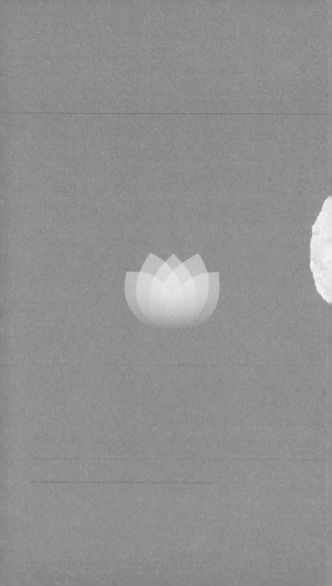

YOGA 365

YOGA 365

DAILY WISDOM FOR LIFE,
ON, AND OFF THE MAT

Susanna Harwood Rubin

CHRONICLE BOOKS
SAN FRANCISCO

Library of Congress Cataloging-in-Publication Data

Names: Rubin, Susanna Harwood.
Title: Yoga 365 : daily wisdom for life, on and off the mat / written and
   illustrated by Susanna Harwood Rubin.
Other titles: Yoga three hundred sixty five
Description: San Francisco : Chronicle Books, [2016]
Identifiers: LCCN 2016023883 | ISBN 9781452145006 (hc : alk.
paper)
Subjects: LCSH: Yoga–Miscellanea.
Classification: LCC B132.Y6 R78 2016 | DDC 181/.45–dc 3 LC
record available at https://lccn.loc.gov/2016023883

Manufactured in China

Design by Allison Weiner
Illustrations by Susanna Harwood Rubin

The information, practices, and poses in this book are not
offered as medical advice or suggested as treatment for any
condition that might require medical attention. To avoid injury,
practice yoga with a skilled instructor and consult a health
professional to determine your body's needs and limitations.
The writer and publisher hereby disclaim any liability from inju-
ries resulting from following any recommendation in this book.

10 9 8 7 6 5 4

Chronicle Books LLC
680 Second Street
San Francisco, California 94107
www.chroniclebooks.com

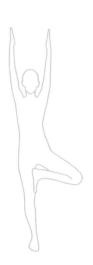

BEGIN IN STABILITY

We build a yoga pose from the ground up in the same way that we would build a house: first, we build a sturdy foundation and then we construct the floors, walls, and roof on top. Without a stable foundation, the structure will not be strong and enduring. Similarly, you need to construct anything in life in this manner, whether it is a friendship, a business, or a creative endeavor. When you begin any endeavor by first establishing stability through communicating, organizing, and goal setting, you give yourself a solid basis on which to build for the future. The next time you embark on a new relationship, job, or project, create a stable base from which to grow. Begin in stability.

MAKE A RESOLUTION TODAY AND AFFIRM IT AGAIN AND AGAIN

Today, resolve to make a change: let go of an old habit that is no longer serving you, or embrace a new habit that will benefit you. Choose a habit that is substantial but small so it is attainable. Practice this resolution daily this week, checking in with yourself at the beginning of each day to focus your intent and at the end of each day to see how you did. Ask yourself: *How did I do today? What was hard? What was easy? Could I support myself better in any way to help me stick with my resolution?* And if you have lapsed, renew your resolution and begin again.

BE POISED
FOR CHANGE

GATE POSE
PARIGHASANA (pa-ree-GAH-sah-nah)

Imagine that in every instant throughout your day, you are at a doorway leading from one moment of your life into the next. With each thought, action, and decision, you step from one moment into another. *Parighasana*, the Sanskrit word for Gate Pose, inspires us to stay steady, grounded, and open as we move through our daily life. *Parigha* is the Sanskrit word for the bar or beam that secures a gate. To form *Parighasana*, kneel on one leg, extend your other leg to the side, reach sideways over the extended leg, and rest your bottom hand on your leg. In doing so, your body takes a shape resembling an open gate. Apply the qualities of Gate Pose to your daily life by being aware of where you are and being open to change.

WE ARE ELEMENTS
OF NATURE

Just like the weather, the seasons, the earth,
and its creatures, we are elements of nature. As
humans, we often see ourselves as being dominant
over nature, using it for its resources in order to
better our lives. The misconception that nature
is there to serve us is at the root of environmental
problems such as pollution and climate change.
The reality is that we are simply elements in a
completely interdependent natural world. What
we do to nature, we do to ourselves. Today, keep
this in mind as you interact with the many elements
of nature around you, and notice how your concept
of yourself in relation to nature shifts and expands.

TELLING YOUR STORY

Imagine you are reading a book in which the actions, habits, and words of the main character are being described by the narrator. Based on what you read, you develop a sense of who that person is and what that person's values are. Similarly, the actions you take and the words you speak tell the people around you the story of *you*. How you behave and conduct yourself in the world is what people know of you. With this in mind, how do you want to interact with the world? Throughout your day today, notice what your actions and words convey about who you are. How are you telling your story?

THE DIVINE IN ME BOWS TO THE DIVINE IN YOU

Namaste (nah-mah-stay)

What is it that makes you want to bow down in awe, gratitude, or reverence? Is it beauty? Kindness? Generosity? When we draw our palms together in prayer and say *Namaste* at the end of a yoga session, we are saying, "The divine in me bows to the divine in you." We say *Namaste* in reverence for what we have just done. We bow to the peace and ease yoga has offered us. We bow to the divine light within us that connects to the greater divine light of yoga.

SPEND TIME WITH OTHERS TO EXPAND YOUR WORLD

People who are different from you can often make good company. Time spent with others can expand your frame of reference so you grow as a person. You become wiser for having entertained ideas that are different from yours, and more tolerant for having been exposed to unfamiliar ways of thinking and being in the world. You have the opportunity to bounce your thinking off of other people and to receive feedback that you wouldn't receive if you only kept your own company. It is through the invigorating friction of difference that we grow as human beings.

MAKE TODAY AN ACT OF CREATIVE SELF-EXPRESSION

Today, infuse your actions and your words with imagination and curiosity, whether you are washing dishes, walking to work, running errands, or making a phone call. Being creative requires approaching everything with a childlike sense of wonder, looking at the world with new eyes, listening with new ears, and responding through these fresh perceptions. When we move through the world in this way, everything we experience becomes richer and more interesting. Our curiosity makes our lives more satisfying because we can become engaged in new and different ways with even the most familiar things around us. Try treating everything you do today with this open attitude. How can you engage in your everyday activities as if you were doing them for the first time? How can you bring a sense of wonder to everything you do so that it becomes newly engaging? Look and act with new eyes so that everything you do today is an expression of your creative self.

FIND YOUR CENTER WHEN THINGS FEEL CHAOTIC

Chaos usually feels like things are scattered, moving in all directions, or shifting unpredictably. When things are chaotic and you need to quiet your mind, it is essential to find your center, that place of balance within yourself, so you can become calm. There are many techniques in yoga that can help you do this. You can close your eyes and meditate, blocking out the external visual world to concentrate on your own inner world. You can observe your breath, offering your attention something simple and powerful on which to focus. You can chant a mantra—or a single word—that calms you. When you need to quiet the raging world outside, these techniques offer you access to your calm center.

WHAT IS
MEDITATION?

Meditation is a conscious interaction between your body and mind that can bring about a state of ease. Meditation practices vary: some invite us to choose a thought, word, object, or sensation on which to focus, so that we can quiet our minds, while others invite us to soften our focus, releasing tension or the mental and emotional clutter within us in order to find equilibrium. Both of these types of meditation can help us create and maintain balance in our lives. We meditate to find peace within our hearts. We meditate to lower our stress levels. We meditate when we need to find focus. When we become adept at our personal meditation practice, we begin to meditate for joy, because over time, meditation becomes blissful. There are infinite ways to meditate because we are all diverse beings with different personalities and needs. Meditation brings balance into our lives and into our hearts. Today, try a new meditation practice and see what it offers you.

BALANCE IS A PROCESS

Finding balance can be thought of as an ongoing process in which your mind and your body converse and negotiate with each other and with the space around you. Your process of finding balance involves the surface on which you sit or stand, the surrounding objects that may support or upset your balance, and your own ever-changing perception of space and stability. As you balance your body on your yoga mat, consider how you might create balance in other parts of your life by accepting that you are in a constant state of process.

YOU ARE POISED
FOR FLIGHT

EAGLE POSE
GARUDASANA (gah-roo-DAH-sah-nah)

In yoga mythology, Garuda is the name of the powerful god Vishnu's companion, whose job is to defend Vishnu and carry him through the skies. Garuda is half-eagle and half-man with enormous wings and a golden crown. Garuda is brave, steady even in the most challenging circumstances, and a powerful warrior. When you wrap arm around arm and leg around leg to balance in *Garudasana*, the Sanskrit name for Eagle Pose, you are invited to find Garuda's qualities within yourself. You can access your power, find and maintain your balance, and do so with elegance and poise.

TREAT YOURSELF WITH COMPASSION

We usually think of compassion as kindness and understanding that we offer to others to support them, but it is equally as important to be compassionate toward ourselves. By treating ourselves with kindness, we can support ourselves and live with greater confidence. Today, practice treating yourself with compassion. If you notice yourself becoming self-critical, try to soften your attitude and your tone toward yourself. If you are feeling tired or stressed out, rest, relax, and do something kind for yourself. How can you best support and love yourself today? How many ways can you find to treat yourself with kindness?

HONOR YOUR BODY

Your body is your means of access to the world. It is through your body that you experience sight, sound, touch, smell, and taste. Your body is made up of countless complex systems that collaborate to enable you to move, to laugh, and to experience pleasure. Honor your body by treating these systems with respect and awe. Honor your body's needs by committing to exercise, good grooming habits, and healthy eating. Love your body despite its limitations. Choose to embrace the challenges of living in an embodied state. Honor your body.

GANESHA AND SUBRAHMANYA'S RACE AROUND THE WORLD

One afternoon, Ganesha, the sweet and steadfast elephant-headed deity, was playing in the shadows of the trees with his brother Subrahmanya. In contrast to Ganesha's contemplative nature, Subrahmanya was a warrior: rapid and precise, he moved as quickly as light. Tired of lounging, smelling flowers, and listening to the buzzing of bees, Subrahmanya challenged Ganesha to a race around the world. Wishing to oblige his brother, Ganesha agreed. Subrahmanya vanished so quickly that he left only a trail of dust on the horizon. Ganesha sighed, pressed himself up, walked across the yard, and made a deliberate circle around his parents, the great god Shiva and magnificent goddess Parvati. He then sat back down under the trees and waited. Moments later, Subrahmanya returned, looking toward his parents for approval. But they explained that Ganesha had won the race. He had understood that what was truly important was right in front of him. Our world is right in front of us. It is simply a matter of recognizing it.

LOOK FOR THE DIVINE
IN EVERYONE

As you move through the world today, try the simple but meaningful exercise of looking for the divine in everyone. The divine, which means something different to everyone, is something that inspires us spiritually or that we hold sacred. The divine can be found in nature, in the universe, and in the deep connectivity we all share as living beings. Look for the divine in people you know and love, in acquaintances, in people who challenge you, and in people you don't even know. Sometimes seeing the divine in someone can have as much to do with what is in your own mind and heart as it does with the attributes of the other person. Try this for a day. The more you seek out the divine, the more you will find it.

FACE FORWARD AND OPEN
TO YOUR FUTURE

Consider this: The front of your body—for example, your eyes, the forward reach of your arms, your chest, knees, and the orientation of your feet—represents your vast potential stretching out in front of you. The back of your body, including your vertebrae, your seat, and the heels of your feet, represents where you have come from—the experiences and accomplishments that have formed and supported you and have brought you to where you are right now. The front of the body is associated with taking action, since most of our actions are performed in front of us. So, facing forward, look toward the horizon today. Draw your attention to what can and may await you. Be mindful of your past choices so that they can intelligently inform your new choices. And step into your future.

YOGA IS: FULLNESS

The Sanskrit word *purnata* (POOR-nah-tah) means fullness, a sweet overflowing experience of abundance. When we catch a glimpse of the beauty of life—when we feel, for even a moment, that we are somehow complete—that is *purnata*. We feel this fullness when we are enveloped by love or when we are buoyed up by good fortune. We also experience this fullness when we are content, as if there were nothing we need that we do not have at that particular moment. Beauty can inspire the experience of *purnata*—art, nature, or anything that fills our hearts and makes us feel whole. When we practice yoga, we can sometimes experience this fullness. Yoga offers us the experience of *purnata*.

THERE IS NO SUCH THING AS INACTION

Whatever you are doing right now—even if you are simply relaxing—you are engaged in some form of action. Consider that inaction is actually a type of action, and that each of our actions is the result of our choosing to perform it. For example, whether you are sitting and staring into space or engaged in a focused activity, you have made a choice to do so. So own your actions—all of them. Today, choose to be fully engaged in whatever it is that you are doing. Throughout the day, ask yourself: *Am I fully engaged in my current action? How might my current activity benefit me?* Then, if you find that a particular action doesn't benefit you, try choosing a different action that does.

CHOOSE HAPPINESS AND MAKE IT A PRACTICE

Sometimes happiness comes easily, but other times it does not. For many of us, happiness emerges from a commitment to experiencing happiness. In times when happiness seems elusive, remember that everything takes practice. First, happiness must be a choice. Once that choice is made, it must then become a practice. When it is our practice, we choose it again and again. We commit to it daily. The choices we make in our lives and the people with whom we choose to surround ourselves should support our happiness. Choose happiness and make it a practice.

CULTIVATE ABUNDANCE IN YOUR LIFE

Cultivate abundance in your life by opening your eyes to the abundance all around you. If you are focusing on all the things you don't have, or on all the ways you aren't achieving what you hope to, or if you are feeling unloved, you are applying a mindset of scarcity rather than one of abundance. When you feel yourself slipping into that mindset, stop. What is that mindset doing for you? Nothing positive. If you focus on scarcity, scarcity is what you will find. Foster feelings of abundance in your life, focusing on what you *do* have. Try to be abundant in your mind, in your heart, and in your attitude in order to draw abundance toward you.

MEDITATE ON A SINGLE POINT TO FIND FOCUS

When our minds are difficult to manage, we have a hard time dropping into a meditative state. We may experience "monkey mind," when our minds leap all over the place. One way to alleviate monkey mind is to choose a single point on which to focus, such as the tip of a candle flame, a small object, or a knot in a wood floor. To practice this type of meditation, choose a focal point directly in front of you, and soften your eyes so that everything around your focal point fades away. Feel the rise and fall of your breath and let it support your focus. With your eyes relaxed but focused, your mind can disengage from mental distractions and release into a calm, meditative state.

STAY PRESENT IN THE MOMENT WHEN THINGS GET TOUGH

When things get tough, choose to stay present in every moment, which will help you stay calm. Invite each breath you take to be a new beginning. Try this: Inhale deeply, filling your body with the energy of your breath. Now exhale, releasing the breath fully and saying to yourself, *Right now, in this moment, I am fine*. Take in another deep breath, and repeat as you exhale, *Now, in this moment, I am fine*. Repeat this process as many times as you need to when things are tough and you want to center yourself. Focusing on the breath in this way helps you stay present in the moment and access calm.

THE MYTH OF KRISHNA
AND KALIYA

Once in the village where the young god Krishna
lived, a giant, poisonous, multi-headed serpent
named Kaliya took up residence in the lake, causing
the waters to become toxic. To help the villagers,
Krishna leapt into the lake to battle with the
serpent, and vanished. After several minutes, the
lake's surface began to ripple and the villagers
saw Krishna rising into the air, playing his flute and
dancing on the back of the serpent. Kaliya swayed
beneath Krishna's feet, intoxicated by his music.
Finally Kaliya said, "I am sorry that I have caused
such destruction, but I am a serpent and it is my
nature to be poisonous." Krishna asked him to
move off into the ocean where his toxicity would
be diluted, and so Kaliya did. Kaliya, the villagers,
and the lake had been in a state of misalignment.
Similarly, when we are in a state of misalignment,
the effects can be toxic. Yoga draws us back into
alignment: body, mind, and heart.

OUR BREATH IS OUR CONVERSATION WITH THE WORLD

Through our breath, we connect to the world around us. When we inhale, the world rushes into our lungs. When we exhale, we offer our breath back out into the world. Our breathing is an intimate interaction with our surroundings, like a meaningful exchange with a loved one. There is a give and take, an absorption and a response. With each complete breath, we take in what is around us, assimilate what nourishes us, and release what we don't need. Our breath is our constant conversation with the world.

COMMIT TO FIVE MINUTES OF YOGA A DAY TO CREATE A HOME PRACTICE

We often put off our home yoga practice because we think that it's not worth doing unless it is substantial, which to many practitioners means a solid hour on our mats. In this way, because we are often pressed for time, or find it difficult to discipline ourselves, we set ourselves up for failure. Try this: Today, take five minutes to do your yoga practice session. And take five minutes again tomorrow. And so on. By committing to five minutes, the idea of a daily practice becomes less daunting. There will be some days in which you keep going beyond five minutes because it feels good, because you have extra time, or because you feel particularly disciplined. And on most days, you can easily meet your basic goal of five minutes and feel a sense of accomplishment, empowering yourself through the daily rhythm of your commitment.

WHAT INSPIRES YOU?

What do you encounter in your daily life that inspires you? Think carefully. What is it that generates ideas and helps motivate you? We can be elevated or crushed by the simplest exchange or the smallest occurrence, so notice what positively shifts your mood or buoys you up, and do your best to connect with at least one of those moments today. If you feel dragged down by anything, remind yourself of one of those positive moments. Reconnect with that feeling of inspiration in your body and mind, like a surge of energy or a cascade of ideas, and invite it to the surface again.

CREATE BALANCE WITH YOUR BODY AND MIND

HEADSTAND POSE
SIRSASANA (sheer-SHAH-sah-nah)

When your body is settled, your heart and mind often are settled as well. *Sirsasana*, the Sanskrit term for Headstand Pose, can settle the body and bring about a feeling of calm. To practice this yoga pose, place the top of your head on the ground, shifting your weight slightly toward your forehead, and place your hands on the ground in front of you to form a triangle with three points of balance. Then, bend your knees to your chest and extend your legs to the sky. Be active rather than passive as you gently press your head and hands into the ground. The pose may seem precarious, but it can actually be very solid. The weight of your head grounds and anchors you, offering a feeling of balance throughout your body.

WRITE TO
RELEASE

One of the best ways to clear your head mentally and emotionally is to write down your thoughts. The writing doesn't have to be beautiful, precise, or clear. Think of the writing as a candid conversation you are having with yourself that will enable you to reveal and then release any upsetting thoughts or mental clutter. Today, try releasing something that is troubling you through a quick five-minute writing session. Write any time: first thing in the morning, during a work break, or before bed. Write without censoring yourself or fixing spelling or grammar. The point is to draw thoughts and feelings out of your body and mind, and to release them onto the page. The practice of writing to release is like taking a mental shower, so that your day and your sleep become cleaner and clearer.

WHEN JUDGMENT SERVES US AND WHEN IT DOESN'T

Throughout each day, we make judgments: what to wear, where to eat, with whom we do and don't wish to engage. We make decisions and judgment calls at our jobs and in every aspect of our personal lives. This behavior can sometimes turn into negativity and needless criticism. While it is healthy and natural to make basic judgments, it is not healthy to create a pattern of critiquing others. We can be selective without condemning. We can say no to others without labeling them as lesser or wrong. Today, watch for moments when your healthy personal judgments begin to shift into criticism or critique. Simply remind yourself that such critical thoughts can be an unnecessary use of your energy and choose to shift your attention to what you do want rather than dwelling on what you don't.

HONOR YOUR HEART'S INTENTION

Anjali Mudra (an-jah-lee MOO-drah)
Mudra of Honoring

Anjali Mudra, a hand gesture in which we draw our palms together in gratitude or in prayer, signifies honoring, and is based on the idea of a lotus blossom with its petals folded together. To form this gesture, hold your hands up in front of you, palms facing each other. Connect your thumbs, your pinkies, your index fingers, your ring fingers, and finish by connecting your middle fingers, the center of the flower. The lotus represents your heart, and when we join our palms in *Anjali Mudra*, we draw our prayers from the depths of our hearts out into the world where we can actualize them. At the beginning and the end of our yoga or meditation session, we draw our hands together in *Anjali Mudra* in gratitude for our practice and to honor our hearts' intentions.

LET GO OF THE PAST TO MOVE FORWARD

If we want to move forward in our lives, we need to let go of the past. When we cling too tightly to defunct concepts of who we are, we hold ourselves back from the new opportunities available to us. We can become stuck in stale conceptions of our identities, which can prevent us from growing and changing. While we need to learn from our past choices and mistakes, we also need to move on from them. What can you relinquish about your past today that will help open you to your future?

KARMA MEANS
ACTION

Every action you take sets into motion a chain
of events. No matter how big or small an action
is, it has an effect: from brushing your teeth
to making a difficult phone call, from making a
big life change to simply walking a different way
to work. The Sanskrit word *karma* (KAR-mah)
means action, and is used to indicate the process
of cause and effect. Although you cannot predict
exactly what will happen as a result of an action
you take, because life also involves chance and
serendipity, if you thoughtfully take action toward
a particular goal, you increase your odds of receiving a particular outcome. As you move through
your day today, seek to be deliberate in the actions
you take yet open to aligning with their outcomes.

TAP INTO YOUR RESOLVE AND YOUR POWER

CHAIR POSE
UTKATASANA (OOT-kah-TAH-sah-nah)

Utkatasana, the Sanskrit word for Chair Pose, requires an enormous amount of lower body strength because we must support our weight in a challenging position. *Utkatasana* builds power and endurance; we strengthen both our legs and our determination through practicing this pose. Standing upright, connect your legs and feet, and bend deeply at the knees until your thighs are almost parallel with the ground. Reach your hips back, and tuck your sitting bones toward the ground. Lift your arms up over your head, and tap into your resolve and your power.

DEVELOP AN INTIMATE RELATIONSHIP WITH YOUR BODY

What does it mean to develop an intimate relationship with your body? It means that you choose to put aside self-criticism in favor of self-embrace. We live in a society that is all too frequently focused on how we measure up, how we compare to an elusive or impossible physical ideal, and what we can do to achieve bodily change. This type of body idealization and comparison is the enemy of intimacy. Intimacy means a close familiarity, an appreciation, an understanding predicated on deep acceptance and affection. Ask yourself: *Which way of thinking about my body sounds better to me?* Release external ideals about what your body "should be" and begin to cultivate intimacy.

DARE TO BE DIFFERENT

There is only one you, so embrace your uniqueness. We need to coexist with other people's habits, interests, and points of view, but we also need to recognize that our own sensibilities are of equal value. When we feel empowered, we can better allow people their own individual identities as well. The more secure we feel about our ideas and opinions, the more easily we can respect those of other people. Embrace your sensibility, acknowledging its uniqueness. Being different isn't bad; it actually makes the world richer and more interesting. When you stand resolutely in your own identity, you create a space in which others can stand as well.

ACKNOWLEDGING EVERYTHING THAT EXISTS

Om or *Aum*
(ohm)

The mantra of mantras, *Om*, is considered to be the vibrational sound of everything that exists—the great cosmic hum of nature. *Om* is also spelled *Aum*, the sound of the mantra rolling through the mouth from back to front. The sound *A* comes from the back of the throat with the mouth open, the sound *U* is made in the middle of the mouth with the lips almost closed, and *M* is the sound made with closed lips, when the sound of *Aum* is finished and you must open your mouth to begin chanting *Aum* again. You can think of *Aum* as the beginning-middle-end of everything: your day, your yoga practice, your life. In nature, everything is always in a process of growing, stabilizing, and dissolving. When we chant *Aum*, we acknowledge these processes within us, connecting us deeply to nature.

DO YOU WANT TO BE RIGHT OR DO YOU WANT TO BE HAPPY?

In conversation, we are often torn between convincing people of our point of view and creating harmony: being right versus being happy. So ask yourself: *Which is more important to me in this particular situation and in this particular moment? Does my desire to win an argument override my desire to have a collegial relationship with a colleague? Does my need to assert my knowledge or point of view prevent a warm exchange of ideas with a friend or family member?* By refusing to listen or to compromise, we can lose more than we gain. Sometimes it is more important to be happy than it is to be right. You can maintain your beliefs while accepting that others wish to maintain theirs as well.

TRANSITION AND CHANGE ARE THE NATURE OF LIFE

Change is the nature of all things. When we try to stop change, we are fighting nature, and that is a battle we cannot win. Look around you: the seasons change, everything is born and then ages, and we are part of that great moving flow of everything in its perpetual state of transition. When we accept that change is the nature of things, we can become more adept at change ourselves. We become fluent in transitions and skilled at adapting to new circumstances. We move with nature as nature, while embracing the fact that we are part of the unending transformation that is life.

BE AT HOME WHEREVER YOU ARE

Ganesha, the elephant-headed deity of yoga mythology, has an enormous belly because he carries the universe within it. For this reason, wherever he is, he is at home. So ask yourself: *How can I, like Ganesha, feel at home in every moment?* Regardless of our current circumstances, we are right here in this moment. Sitting, standing, or moving through the world, we carry our experience of the world within us. All we have to do is recognize this reality. When we choose to be at home wherever we are, we develop a deep unshakeable sense of belonging everywhere. We are always at home because the world is always with us.

MEDITATE ON
A WORD

First thing in the morning, choose one word that describes what you want from your day. For example, you may wish for strength, compassion, joy, contentment, ease, peace, inspiration, or patience. Write the word down or simply keep it in mind. Throughout your day, repeat it to yourself and consider what it means to you. Keep returning to this word as a reminder and a point of reference. Investigate it. Take note of moments when it reveals itself in the events of your day. Notice when you need it most as a reminder of how you wish to feel today.

LIVING WITH OUR LIMITATIONS

Recognizing our limitations is wise: it can keep us safe from injury or unwise personal and professional decisions, and it gives us a sense of boundaries. But limitations are not prohibitions. If we can embrace our limitations with humor and self-acceptance, we can still enjoy singing even if we are not the best singers, playing a sport just for fun, or dancing for pleasure rather than for performance. Limitations give us perspective, pointing out the ways in which we are gifted as much as the ways in which we may be simply average. And that contrast can help us love who we are, limitations and all.

OPEN YOUR HEART WITH URDHVA DANURASANA

UPWARD-FACING BOW POSE

URDHVA DANURASANA (oor-dvah dan-nur-AH-sah-nah)

Think of all the work you do during the day that constricts the front of your body: sitting, working at a computer, bending forward to listen and to speak, preparing and eating food. *Urdhva Danurasana*, the Sanskrit term for Upward-Facing Bow Pose, also known as Wheel or Backbend, is an opportunity to completely reverse this folded-in sensation and ecstatically open the front of the body. Lie on your back with your hands on the floor by your head, and firmly reach your pelvis and then your heart up to the sky so that you are balancing on your hands and feet. Your body, arched like a bow, reverses any tightness that may have gathered in the front of your body throughout your day, opening your heart and shifting your perspective.

FORGIVE YOURSELF

Take a minute to think about the ways that you chastise or criticize yourself. Ask yourself: *What does this self-criticism do for me? And what is it doing to me?* When you hold on to regret about things you have done, you prevent yourself from growing. Worse, you block yourself from self-love. In effect, you are holding a grudge against yourself. And so you lose doubly in this situation: as the grudge-holder and as the recipient of your own criticism. It doesn't matter how bad what you did may have been. If you have done all you could to rectify the situation, it is time to move on. And moving on only happens through forgiveness. Forgive yourself.

HONOR NATURE TO HONOR YOURSELF

Honor nature. Honor the earth. It is important to remember that you are part of nature, so when you honor it, you also honor yourself. The way you treat nature says something about how you view yourself. When we litter, pollute, and disregard nature, we are disrespecting ourselves as well. Imagine that the landscape in front of you is a vast extension of your body, and just as your body is positively or negatively affected by what you put on it and into it, so is this great landscape. Treat nature as well as you do your own body—with the wonderment, care, and nurturing it deserves. Honor nature to honor yourself.

THE MYTH OF AGNI AND SWAHA

When the entire universe was created, the gods did not yet have enough food. They went to chat with Brahma, the god of creation, about it. Brahma decided that to make sure there was always enough food for the gods, he would have people build and feed fires to honor and feed the gods. Agni, the god of fire, tried to ignite a fire, but couldn't because he was hungry and didn't have enough energy to do so. To help Agni, Brahma transformed Swaha, a seductive nymph, into a full goddess, and married her to Agni. Agni fell madly in love with Swaha's beauty, and as his temperature rose, Agni was able to ignite a fire; the fire burned, and the gods were properly honored and fed. This myth of Agni and Swaha reminds us that we all need inspiration to motivate us in our lives. Ask yourself this: *What energizes me? Who helps me tap into my power?*

YOU ARE BODY.
YOU ARE SPIRIT.

You are body. You are made up of bone and muscle, skin and blood. You move, you eat, you hear, see, and taste the world around you. You take up physical space in the world. You are also spirit. Made of thoughts and dreams, feelings and intuitions, you are more than just the sum of your physical parts. Your body houses your spirit, and your spirit supports and sustains your body. There is no need to separate the two or value one over the other, because they are inextricably intertwined. Love your body. Love your spirit. You are both.

FINDING EASE WITH OTHERS

We want to be at ease in the world. We want to be comfortable enough in our own skin that we can enjoy the company of others—their differences and their opinions. When we cultivate ease within ourselves, we find ease in our interactions with others. Notice if you are worrying excessively about what others think of you. This is often at the root of any discomfort in social situations. Remind yourself that your thoughts and feelings are as important as anyone else's, and that, in all likelihood, there is someone else in the room who feels just as you do. Then, take in a deep breath and, on the exhale, release the anxiety, the second-guessing of your-self, and the very notion that others' opinions are in any way more significant than yours. In this way, you create the space for ease.

YOGA IS:
HOLISTIC

ga's power resides in its ability to impact our
...nds, our bodies, and our hearts. While we may
engage in a predominantly physical practice, this
act of joining breath to movement that we call
yoga creates mental and emotional change as well.
Yoga's approach is holistic, inviting these three
key aspects of our existence into conversation
with each other. When our bodies feel healthy and
vibrant, our minds and hearts often follow suit.
Inversely, when we feel spacious in our minds and
hearts, our bodies often open up as well. Yoga
addresses our whole complex selves.

CONNECT WITHIN TO FIND COURAGE

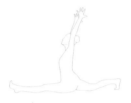

SPLIT POSE
HANUMANASANA (hah-noo-mah-NAH-sah-nah)

In yoga mythology, the monkey god Hanuman leaps through the air to courageously defend those he loves. *Hanumanasana*, also known as Split Pose, invites you to courageously connect with what you love. In this challenging pose, which requires that your lower body be thoroughly warmed up before attempting it, you engage the muscles of your legs and around your pelvis in order to safely arrange yourself in a split position. This muscular engage-ment offers an overall sense of connectivity in your body and consequently in your heart. Strengthened by this connectivity, you—like Hanuman—can leap courageously toward what you love and want in your life.

OUR DIFFICULT EMOTIONS HAVE A PURPOSE

While we may not enjoy experiencing anger, sadness, fear, or disgust, this range of emotions helps make us complex, empathetic, and empowered individuals. We learn from our negative experiences as well as our positive ones. We decide what we do and do not want in our lives. It is through experiencing sadness that we recognize and appreciate joy. It is through the experience of anger eating away at us that we work for peace. Fear and disgust show us what we wish to turn away from, revealing what we wish to turn toward. Today, seek to notice the emotions you are experiencing, and let them be your teachers, bringing insight and awareness into your heart and mind.

GENEROSITY CREATES POSITIVE ENERGY

When you give to others, you generate positive energy. It doesn't take much to help other people feel good about themselves. Today, try to offer a small act of generosity toward another person. This could be leaving a thoughtful note for someone, giving money to a person in need, offering a compliment, even holding a door open. The gesture may be small but it is a gift that will feel substantial to the person who receives it. For the next week, see if you can continue to offer one act of kindness a day: to a stranger, to a friend, or to a family member. Then check in with yourself and see how your generosity resonates within you as well.

MALA
MEDITATION

A mala is a string of prayer beads that can be used as a meditation tool. A mala helps focus our minds and allows us to count the number of times we repeat a mantra during meditation. To use a mala for meditation, drape it over the last three fingers of your right hand and, beginning at the big bead at the base of the mala, known as the guru or teacher bead, use your thumb to pull each bead down, repeating your mantra out loud or silently every time. You can move once through the beads of the mala or you can choose to switch directions and continue. Mala meditation offers just enough focus and just enough freedom to draw you into a meditative state.

YOUR FACE IS A CANVAS

Your face is the surface on which your thoughts and feelings are often most clearly displayed to the world. While your everyday body language can be highly expressive, it is on your face where your emotions often paint a vivid depiction of your inner condition. Whether you are experiencing anger, sadness, confusion, amusement, or joy, your face has an infinite number of ways to display the nuances of your state of mind. Today, gain self-awareness by noticing the ways in which your face responds to what you are feeling and displays it to the world.

THE MYTH OF SHIVA'S BLUE THROAT

Long ago, a precious elixir of immortality had been hidden in the ocean of consciousness, which contained everything that existed. Hoping to locate the elixir, all the gods and demons joined forces to churn the ocean. Searching for the elixir was a dangerous endeavor, for as they churned the ocean, they risked uncovering all sorts of perils. But they churned nonetheless. Soon, a deadly poison emerged from the ocean. The gods and demons called to Shiva, the greatest of the gods, for help. Unperturbed, Shiva took the poison into his mouth. His wife, the goddess Parvati, lunged toward him, fearing for his life, and grabbed his throat with her hands to prevent him from swallowing it. Held in his throat, the poison turned Shiva's throat blue but did not harm him. From that day forward, he was referred to as the Blue-Throated One. This myth asks us: *How might we experience difficulties in our lives without letting them harm us? How can we maintain our strength and equilibrium in the face of our greatest challenges?*

OBSERVE YOUR BREATH

Your breath is like an ocean: vast and ever flowing. There are times when it is rapidly moving and tumultuous, and times when it is soft and smooth. Your breath can be forceful and loud or it can be so light as to be inaudible. By varying in this way, your breath tells a story of each moment. Your breath's ability to calm and soothe teaches you the value of slowness to create ease. Your breath's depth offers you the experience of expansiveness. Your inhaling and exhaling remind you of the rise and fall of everything in life. Focusing on your breath can calm you, energize you, and offer you a sense of the wonder of your own body. Today, pause several times and observe your breath.

SAY YES
TO LIFE

Whatever is going on in our lives, moving on our mats enlivens our bodies, eases our minds, and enables us to more readily access our hearts. On any given day, yoga makes us feel peaceful, energized, or simply happy. The exploratory nature of our yoga practice can make us curious about our bodies. The problem-solving challenge of a particular pose engages our effort and our attention. Yoga helps us live more fully and deeply, making us excited about life. By saying yes to yoga, we say yes to life. Roll out your mat, step onto it, and begin to move.

WHEN YOU BELIEVE IN YOURSELF, YOU BECOME FEARLESS

Abhaya Mudra (a-BHAI-ya MOO-drah)
Mudra of Fearlessness

How would it feel to believe in yourself so fiercely that you follow your dreams, not letting anyone or anything lessen your faith in yourself? Undeterred, you pursue what you want and what you love without hesitation. You don't let fear hold you back or self-doubt undermine your aspirations. *Abhaya Mudra* is a hand gesture that represents fearlessness. To form this mudra, lift your right forearm so that your palm faces out. This simple yet powerful gesture symbolizes your fearless commitment to yourself, and invites others to commit to fearlessness as well.

YOUR ENVIRONMENT TELLS A STORY ABOUT WHO YOU ARE

Look around you. The environment you have created for yourself tells a story of who you are. Whether you live a pared-down existence with only the necessities, surround yourself with objects holding sentimental value, or design your personal space to express a particular aesthetic, the way in which you choose, arrange, and organize your surroundings is a reflection of your values and life choices. As you look, ask yourself: *What do my choices tell me about myself?* Invite the environment that you have created to mirror insights about your personality and values back to you. Recognize it as a storyteller in your life narrative.

ACKNOWLEDGE YOUR WEAKNESSES TO EMBRACE YOUR STRENGTHS

By examining our weaknesses as well as our strengths, we are better able to understand ourselves, thereby knowing when we need help or guidance, and knowing when we are capable of offering similar assistance to others. Our vulnerabilities and frailties illuminate by contrast our gifts and strengths. Through a full recognition of our strengths and weaknesses, we become aware of our knowledge and power, and aware of when we need to enlist the knowledge and power of others in order to achieve our goals. This self-knowledge enables us to use the strengths we possess to move forward and offer our best selves to the world. Acknowledge your weaknesses in order to embrace your strengths.

TAKE A LEAP TOWARD YOUR DREAM

What do you dream of doing in your life? What do you really want? Without excessive analyzing or self-doubt, take action on this quest today. Begin by making yourself a list of action items. Ask yourself: *What concrete steps can I take today, tomorrow, and the next day to move toward making my dream a reality?* Make a phone call, send an e-mail, change a habit. Instead of sitting and pondering the pros and cons of a particular action, simply do it. Your action may or may not move you closer to your dream, but if you do nothing, you have no chance of success. Increase your odds of attaining your dream. The time to begin is now.

BE PROUD OF WHO YOU ARE

ONE-LEGGED KING PIGEON POSE
EKA PADA RAJAKAPOTASANA
(eh-kah PAH-dah RAH-jah-kah-poh-TAH-sah-nah)

Picture a pigeon's full, rounded chest of iridescent feathers gleaming in the sun. While pigeons are often considered to be ordinary birds, they hold themselves proudly. Hold yourself proudly in *Eka Pada Rajakapotasana*, the Sanskrit name for One-Legged King Pigeon Pose. *Eka* means one, *pada* means leg or foot, *raja* means king, and *kapota* means pigeon. From Downward-Facing Dog Pose, slide one knee forward and out to the side, extend your other leg behind you, and lower your pelvis to the ground. Bend your back knee and reach back for your foot with one or both hands. Open your chest toward the sky like a pigeon, then lift your heart fully, expressing pride in who you are.

YOUR HANDS, YOUR TOUCH, YOUR ENGAGEMENT WITH THE WORLD

Using your hands is one of the main ways you interact with the world. Take a moment right now to think of how much you have already done with your hands today: pushing, pulling, opening, arranging, lifting. Your hands are powerful but can also perform delicate and intricate tasks. When you touch another person with your hands, the way in which you touch is a form of communication. You can touch roughly or gently, tentatively or confidently, harshly or in a loving manner. This message is also true of how you place your hands on your own body. Today, draw your awareness to the ways in which you offer touch and notice how it impacts you and others.

EACH YOGA POSE INVITES YOU TO EXPERIENCE YOURSELF

Every time you move your body into a yoga pose, you have the opportunity to experience yourself in a specific way, because each pose taps into a particular aspect of who you are. If it is a pose that you love, you may connect with your calm or energized self, or perhaps your curious or intrigued self. With a pose that is challenging for you, you may experience your frustrated, perplexed, or perhaps humorous self. The next time you practice yoga, try to receive each pose as an experience of yourself. Through your practice, your self-knowledge will grow and deepen.

I BOW DOWN TO THE GREAT CREATIVE POWER OF THE UNIVERSE

Om Shri Matre Namaha
(ohm shree mah-tray nah-mah-ha)

For connection and support, we chant *Om Shri Matre Namaha*. *Om* evokes everything that exists. *Shri* means auspicious, abundant, and life-affirming. *Matre* refers to the divine mother. *Namaha* means that we bow down, we honor. When we chant *Om Shri Matre Namaha*, we call to the maternal pro-creative power that exists in the universe; to the energy through which we were created, born, and continue to be nurtured and sustained; to the great mother who holds us in the abundance of her embrace. This power is present whenever we need solace, whenever we feel the need to be spiritually held.

APPRECIATING CONNECTION

Which people do you connect with in your life? Notice who they are and what qualities they possess. They might be very similar to you or very different from you, but there is something between you that resonates, some question that is answered through the relationship, some need that is met in some way. If they are similar to you, it might be because you understand each other easily. If you are different from them, it may be that you complement each other. Friendship and chemistry are somewhat mysterious, but strive to appreciate your friends for their similarities and for their differences; the similarities will offer you understanding and the differences will offer you fresh perspectives into yourself.

ALIGN YOUR ACTIONS
WITH YOUR WORDS

Sometimes our actions contradict our words,
conveying who we would like to be rather than who
we actually are. For example, we may say that we
value something, but our actions suggest that we
actually do not value it. When we recognize this
contradiction, we get to know ourselves better, and
we can choose whether we want to continue living
in contradiction or change our behavior so that it
better illustrates our words. Today, ask yourself:
*Are my actions aligned with my words? How can
I create and maintain a consistency between my
actions and my words in my daily life?* Then try
moving through your day in a way that develops
and supports an aligned integrity between what
you say and what you do.

HOLD THE SPACE
FOR OTHERS

When people we care for need support or need
to feel safe, we are given an opportunity to hold
the space for them. What does "hold the space"
mean? It means listening and offering a peaceful
place in which the person can talk, cry, or simply
sit in silence. Holding the space is not always
easy. You have to be calm, strong in your caring
for that person, and allow that person the freedom
to do what he or she needs to do. You create a
healing field in which they can sit or wander until
they are ready to move on. When we hold the
space for others, we honor them, and we become
our best selves.

MEDITATE BY SERVING OTHERS

Serving others can be a form of meditation. The Sanskrit word for this is *seva* (SAY-vah), meaning selfless service. Engaging in *seva* can be anything from doing volunteer work to choosing a day in which you focus on helping the people you encounter. Today, see if you can engage in *seva* by offering to help people in small but substantial ways. If someone drops something, pick it up and hand it back to him or her. Offer someone your seat. Reach out to someone who needs a kind word or some support. Clean or straighten up a work or home space for someone else. See how many of these small acts of kindness you can offer. The point of *seva* is to access your generosity and offer it to the world.

TAKE YOURSELF ON A DATE

Today, whether you are single or in a relationship, make a date with yourself. Treat yourself to something special just like you would treat another person you care for. Engage in an activity that you can thoroughly enjoy alone. Go to a museum. Go for a walk in nature. Wander through the city. Sit and people watch. Take yourself to lunch or to dinner— a really good one. And enjoy your own company the way you would enjoy the company of someone with whom you are madly in love. Listen to your thoughts; admire and compliment yourself. Today, make a date with yourself. Lavish yourself with attention and love.

ROOT DOWN AND BALANCE YOURSELF

HANDSTAND POSE (OR UPSIDE-DOWN TREE POSE)
ADHO MUKHA VRKSASANA
(ah-doh moo-kah vri-KSHAH-sah-nah)

Imagine a tree with enormous limbs and branches. Now imagine you could see beneath the ground to the root structure that mirrors the web of branches aboveground. *Adho Mukha Vrksasana* means Upside-Down Tree Pose in Sanskrit, and is more commonly known as Handstand Pose. When you practice Handstand Pose, your hands create your foundation like the roots of a tree, supporting your body as it reaches toward the sky. This yoga pose reminds us that we always can find ways in which to root down and balance ourselves no matter how precarious the circumstances.

BE EMPATHETIC, BUT ACT WITH COMPASSION

The two words empathy and compassion are often used interchangeably, but there is a difference between them. Empathy is stepping into another person's shoes, feeling what they feel, or even taking on whatever they are feeling. Compassion is seeing and comprehending in a supportive manner what another person is experiencing. While empathy allows us to deeply understand others, it can compromise our well-being when it leads us to take on their emotional state. In contrast, when we practice compassion, we maintain our own well-being, which lets us be better equipped to assist others. Today, try offering compassion toward someone who needs it in the form of supportive words or actions.

HONOR YOUR TEACHERS

Think of everyone you have ever learned from: your family members, schoolteachers, friends—anyone who has ever guided you in some way. Then consider what you have learned from people who have challenged or wronged you. All are your teachers. Some may have offered tough life lessons by demonstrating how you don't want to act in the world. Others may have opened doors for you that you didn't know were there. Give thanks, because all of these people—supportive and difficult, thoughtful and cruel, inspiring and frustrating—have brought you to where you are right now. Honor the wisdom they have helped you gain, and think about how you can use it to move forward in your life.

THE MYTH OF BABY KRISHNA AND THE DUST DEMON

In the town where the baby god Krishna lived, there was a demon who was fixated on kidnapping the powerful young god. When Krishna's mother had put him down for a moment, the demon Trinavarta transformed himself into a powerful dust storm that obscured everyone's vision. Krishna's mother, Yashoda, caught a glimpse of Krishna as he was whisked away into the sky, and then, losing sight of him, she collapsed. Flying through the air, Krishna laughed, because he was assured and centered in his power as a god. He knew the demon was no match for him. He steadily made himself heavier and heavier until Trinavarta was overcome. Once he weighed him down, Krishna grabbed the demon by the neck and drew him back down to the ground. When the dust cleared and Yashoda sat up, she saw baby Krishna happily playing while seated on the vanquished demon's chest. Krishna shows us that when we are centered in who we are, and assured and steady in our own power, we cannot be defeated.

YOU ARE A WORLD
UNTO YOURSELF

Just as the world is made up of many parts—
different lands, bodies of water, plants, animals,
and people—you are made up of many varied
interdependent parts. Like the world, your body
is a complex ecosystem that is perpetually shifting
and adjusting in response to its changing environment. And just as your organs, bones, fluids, and
breath are a part of your personal ecosystem, your
body is a component of the world's ecosystem. You
are simultaneously unique and part of a greater
whole. You are a world unto yourself, yet you are
connected to everything that exists.

KNOW WHEN TO ENGAGE
AND WHEN TO LET GO

There are times when you need to stand up for what you believe. At these times, you might engage in a conflict that ultimately leads to greater under-standing. There are other times, however, when it is best to walk away, seeing that the discussion cannot possibly have a productive outcome. Some-times disagreement helps lead to positive change, but other times it can do more harm than good. The next time you find yourself in a disagreement, ask yourself: *Can compromise or understanding result from this discussion?* If not, letting go may be the wisest decision.

YOGA IS:
ALIGNMENT

Yoga aligns body, mind, and heart. But to experience this degree of alignment, we may need to begin by finding alignment within our own bodies. When we start a yoga practice, we begin to understand our bodies more fully: the ways they move and their particular challenges and limitations. Once we gain a certain level of insight, we can develop a conscious bodily alignment that serves us, from protecting our joints and spine to noticing where we are tight or where we store tension. When we align our bodies in a healthier way, we begin to thrive.

FIND BALANCE
TO FIND PEACE

PEACEFUL WARRIOR POSE
VIPARITA VIRABHADRASANA
(vi-pa-REE-tah VI-rah-bah-DRA-sah-nah)

Finding peace is not always easy—sometimes you have to strive for it like a warrior. Standing steadily in *Viparita Virabhadrasana*, the Sanskrit name for Peaceful Warrior Pose or Reverse Warrior Pose, your legs are spread apart, with your front knee bent and your back foot fully rooted to the ground. Arch your torso back while extending one arm and resting your other hand on your back leg. With your lower body leaning forward while your upper body leans back, you embody the physical process of give and take—of balance-seeking. Finding peace often entails finding a balance between the aggressive and receptive parts of ourselves. Be a warrior for peace. Be firm in your resolve and then open to receive.

LOOK FOR LIFE'S SWEETNESS

What is your outlook when you enter a room? Do you look for something interesting, inspiring, or beautiful? Do you look for life's sweetness? Or do you immediately begin critiquing what you see? It is easy to fall into a pattern of criticizing and reacting negatively, but it is important to realize that this is a choice and that you can change it. If you have to choose between focusing on negative qualities and focusing on sweetness, why would you choose anything but sweetness? When we look for life's sweetness, we find it. That is not to say that everything is sweet, or that we shouldn't speak out when it isn't. But in an everyday sense, ask yourself at any given moment: *What can I find here that is sweet? How can I invite that experience of sweetness more deeply into my life?*

TRUST THE
UNIVERSE

What does it mean to trust the universe? We don't know what will happen to us in life, but we know we are part of a complex system of interconnectivity. Whatever may happen, we are deeply woven into the fabric of the entire universe. So when you feel alone, when you feel alienated, when you feel lesser than, remember this: There is nowhere else you need to be and nobody else who you need to be. You are never alone. You are fine as you are. You are right here, cradled in the arms of the universe, just like the rest of us.

MAKE YOUR MORNING INTO
A MEDITATIVE RITUAL

Today, bring a meditative focus to each part of your morning ritual in order to appreciate your daily life. To do this, simply bring mindfulness to each action that you take, from the way you get out of bed to the personal habits and activities you engage in before you leave home. Keep your mind on exactly what you are doing at every moment. If you are washing yourself, notice the feeling of water on your skin. While you prepare and eat your breakfast, direct an easy attentiveness to the process, taking pleasure in each movement and step of the preparation and eating. Extend this attention and care to everything you do this morning, setting a focused and mindful tone for the events of the rest of your day.

CREATE THE SACRED

Anything around you can be sacred. An object is sacred because of the context in which it exists. If a flower is on the ground outside, it is simply a beautiful part of nature. But when that flower is placed on a home altar or given as a gift, it takes on a different meaning because of where it is placed or the spirit in which it is given. A conversation can be sacred if the intention, care, and trust are there. Sacred can mean valued, holy, something that you designate as worthy of your veneration. Through your choices and commitment, you have the capacity to create the sacred in your everyday life.

THE MYTH OF GANESHA
AND GAJAMUKHA

Ganesha and Gajamukha were identical-looking
beings who had elephant heads and round, heavy
human bodies. Ganesha had received his head as
a gift from his father and uncles, so he felt joyful
about his looks since they were given to him in
love. Gajamukha had received his head as a curse
from the gods because of his bad behavior, so he
felt bitter about his looks since they were imposed
upon him in anger. One day, when Gajamukha was
feeling particularly resentful, he convinced the
reluctant Ganesha to participate in a wrestling
match. The two huge creatures slammed into each
other and began grappling. Ganesha gracefully
evaded Gajamukha's grasp, moving so rapidly that
he pinned Gajamukha to the earth in a few minutes.
Defeated, Gajamukha felt his anger drain from him,
and asked Ganesha, "How are you so heavy yet
so graceful? How do you move so joyfully in your
body?" Ganesha told him, "You must accept who
you are and love yourself." Contentment and joy
are states of mind that begin with acceptance and
self-love.

CONNECT YOUR MIND TO YOUR HEART THROUGH YOUR BREATH

Take a deep inhale, envisioning your breath flowing directly into your mind and heart. On your exhale, imagine any tension in your mind and heart floating away. By releasing this tension, you cultivate an openness that enables a connection between your mind, the center of your analytical intelligence, and your heart, the center of your emotional intelligence. On your next inhale, deepen this connection between these two powerful areas of yourself. On your next exhale, relax into the sweetness of this connection. Feel the rise and fall of your breath creating the experience of connectivity between your analytical self and your emotional self, between your mind and your heart.

RELEASE CONTROL TO COLLABORATE WITH THE UNIVERSE

We cannot control everything. Sometimes we need to step back and let things unfold as they will. We can try to direct the outcomes of our actions, but at a certain point, we need to let play out what we have set in motion. We need to release a bit of control. Giving up control can actually be a relief—it is an admission that we are not the only force in the universe, and that, in fact, we are one force in conversation with many other forces, from the forces of nature to the energy and interests of the people around us. For example, we cannot force a flower to open its petals and bloom; we must wait for it to open in its own time. Similarly, we cannot make a person agree with us; we can just present our thoughts and invite that person to consider them. In addition, when we respect nature's rhythms or listen to another person's ideas, we are given an opportunity to grow and learn. We are in a collaborative relationship with everything that exists. And we can try to give and receive within this collaboration.

YOGA IS: MOVING MEDITATION

Today, consider your yoga practice as a form of moving meditation. You step onto your mat and invite your body to move, guided by your breath. You apply form and alignment to your body, releasing yourself into the vibrant rhythm that results. Your mat is your delineated meditation space as your body moves from pose to pose, shape to shape, with each movement and each breath. Relaxed but focused, you find the deep calm emerging from sustained deliberate movement. You let your body take the lead and it draws you into a flowing meditative state.

ALL IS OKAY IN THIS MOMENT. AND THIS MOMENT. AND THIS MOMENT.

Affirm your life in every minute. Be mindful of the past and open to the future, but when the past feels undermining or the future overwhelming, choose to be fully in the present. When we spend too much time agonizing about past mistakes, we lose track of what is happening right before us. When we are overly anxious about what is to come, we lose the joy of living our daily lives. Try this: Ask yourself, *Is this particular moment okay?* Then affirm, *Yes, this moment is okay. And now, this moment is also okay. And now this one.* When you feel yourself losing your connection to the moment, ask yourself this question and then answer it again and again.

HOLD YOURSELF IN MEDITATION

Dhyana Mudra (dee-YAH-nah MOO-drah)
Mudra of Contemplation

Dhyana Mudra is the mudra, or hand gesture, signifying *dhyana*, the Sanskrit term for a meditative state. Resting your hands in your lap, right hand cradled in the left and palms facing up, touch your thumbs, lifting them slightly over the palms as if you were carefully holding something precious. Your hands represent your body, creating a container for your meditation. As your hands come together, close your eyes and allow yourself to feel held in the gentle but powerful embrace of your meditation practice.

BALANCE IS A JUGGLING OF ASYMMETRIES

Balance is a juggling of asymmetries in our bodies as well as in our lives. When we stand on one foot in a yoga pose, we are creating a radical asymmetry in our bodies, yet we can find balance within that asymmetry: we shift a hip or a shoulder, we engage muscles, and root down to make contact with the ground beneath us. Finding balance makes our asymmetries exciting and beautiful. In our lives, things rarely happen exactly as planned: we are frequently thrown off balance and have to change, be flexible, and negotiate with ourselves and with others to find balance once again. If you find that you are off-balance, consider that you are simply positioned to find your balance again in a new way.

CREATE THE STORY
OF YOUR LIFE

We create our life narrative. Every decision we make initiates another chapter in our lives. While we can't control everything that happens to us, we can take charge of writing as much of our story as possible. Take action. Own your mistakes. Do your best. We are creative beings, and every single day offers us the opportunity to begin again. Invite today to be an artistic project in which you take creative chances without fear or hesitation. If your life is a story and you are the protagonist, how do you want the narrative of today to read? Do the writing today to create the story of your life.

YOGA IS:
MIND + BODY + HEART

The Sanskrit word *yoga* means to yoke: to join or connect. We choose to practice yoga because it does more than simply stretch and strengthen our bodies. We practice yoga because we are seeking the experience of connecting our bodies more fully to our minds and hearts. Yoga offers us this experience of connectivity. Over the course of a yoga practice session, the opening of our bodies triggers a similar opening in our minds and a consequent opening of our hearts. In this place of openness, we are able to experience a deep sense of connectivity, linking these three essential parts of who we are.

CULTIVATE INNER STRENGTH TO ACCESS YOUR INNER COURAGE

To thrive, we need courage. It takes courage to listen to our inner voice urging us to look at something challenging within ourselves no matter how difficult that may be. At other times, we need courage to look at one of life's tough realities that we need to accept inwardly. To access this courage, we need the inner strength that we cultivate through meditation and yoga. These practices develop and strengthen us from the inside, so that we will have the courage to address our personal challenges within and without.

STAND IN YOUR GREATNESS

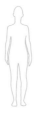

MOUNTAIN POSE
TADASANA (tah-DAH-sah-nah)

Can you own your greatness? Your greatness is the accumulation of all aspects of your personality: your strengths, weaknesses, skills, and challenges, mixed together to form the unique being that is you. *Tadasana* is the Sanskrit name for Mountain Pose. When you stand in *Tadasana*, chest open, arms by your sides, feeling your body reach from the ground into the air, you assert your singularity and remember your immensity. If you find that you chronically self-criticize or denigrate your accomplishments, you are denying your greatness. Step into this yoga pose inspired by the majesty of a mountain and recognize the greatness within you.

DECLUTTER YOUR ENVIRONMENT TO DECLUTTER YOUR LIFE

It is challenging to think and work when our environments are in a state of disorder. External clutter often mirrors internal clutter. Notice if you find it difficult to get things done when your surroundings are disordered. For a greater sense of order and peace of mind, address the stacks and clean up the dust. Throw out what you don't need. If you thrive in a minimal, uncluttered environment, devote time to maintaining that each day. If you love surrounding yourself with objects and books, arrange them artfully. Notice how, when your life gets crazy, your surroundings become disordered. A peaceful environment makes us feel peaceful. An uncluttered environment offers us clarity.

YOU MIRROR THE UNIVERSE

You are a part of the universe. You are a microcosm of a greater reality. And just like the universe, you are vast and complex, always revealing different aspects of yourself at every moment. Like the universe, you are a body of complex systems and relationships with certain distinct qualities yet ever changing. You possess constellations of talents, gifts, and characteristics. You are a creative force that forms order and makes change. You act and are acted upon by everything around you. You mirror the universe.

FIND YOUR INNER STRENGTH

Om Dum Durgaye Namaha
(ohm doom door-gah-yay nah-mah-hah)

In yoga mythology, Durga is a fearless warrior goddess who vanquishes demons. Her mantra tells us to face our fears, stand up for what we believe in, and bravely engage in the world. She is our inner strength itself. *Om* evokes everything that exists. *Dum* is Durga's "seed syllable," meaning it contains her power in the way that an acorn contains an oak tree. *Durgaye* is how we sing her name in the mantra, and *Namaha* means that we bow down, we honor. When we chant *Om Dum Durgaye Namaha*, we call upon the pure strength that resides within us, and we step into our power.

CHANCE ENCOUNTERS CAN TRANSFORM OUR LIVES

Sometimes people enter our life at a particular time for a particular reason. They may be disruptive or soothing, they may help us or challenge us, but regardless, they get us to a new place. Sometimes we need to be disrupted and other times we need assistance or support, and we may encounter just the right person to help us make that shift, whether it concerns an exciting new life decision or the realization that we need to let something go. The person may remain in our life or may vanish, but we can be grateful for their having been a catalyst for growth and change. If there is someone who has recently served this purpose for you, offer that person gratitude for helping you grow.

CULTIVATING YOUR INNER VOICE

Today, listen carefully to the ways in which you speak to yourself, so you can examine your inner conversation. Ask yourself: *Is it helpful? Is it honest? Is it kind? Or is it defeatist, dishonest, or critical?* It is possible to change your inner conversation. First, listen, notice, and even record the things you hear yourself thinking about yourself and about others. Try spending a day taking note of your thoughts. At the end of the day, look at your patterns: What is helpful and what is damaging? Decide to rid yourself of whatever is dragging you down. Hold on to what is serving you—what buoys you up and what elevates others. Cultivating your inner voice so that it uplifts your inner and outer life is a transformational practice.

MEDITATE WITH YOUR EYES OPEN

Embrace the world through your eyes. Receive all of the visual information that is presenting itself to you right now. Take it in: the things, the spaces between things, the light, and the shadow. Let the world's visual abundance offer itself to you as if the universe is giving you a gift. Notice the layers of detail that you may often overlook. Gaze upon the infinite textures and colors of whatever is around you. Dedicate your entire mental focus to a visual exploration of what you see in front of you. Let yourself marvel. Allow your sense of wonder to extend to everything that exists, including you. This meditation is a prayer of gratitude to and appreciation for the visible world.

EMBRACING OUR IMPERFECTIONS

Our imperfections are the source of our individuality. What we perceive as our flaws are the particularities that make us distinctive. What we sometimes view as a weakness or an imperfection is actually something that is simply different. Instead of seeing our distinctive qualities as wrong or undesirable, try viewing them as assets. Think of what you love in your friends—the specific quirks that make them stand out, make you laugh, provoke your curiosity, and make them uniquely themselves. Try to view yourself in this same light. Embrace your perceived imperfections as essential aspects of your specialness, your you-ness, your own particular kind of beauty.

STABILIZE TO SUPPORT YOURSELF

CAMEL POSE
USTRASANA (oosh-TRAH-sah-nah)

Ustrasana, the Sanskrit name for Camel Pose, is a backbend that arranges your body into the shape of a camel's hump. Kneeling, arch backward and take hold of your heels, which expands your chest and the front of your rib cage. The kneeling position provides your body with more stability than other backbends in which you might be balancing on your hands or feet. This greater stability means the pose requires less energy, which mirrors how camels—known to be both powerful and gifted at conserving energy—survive in the desert. The energy conserved in Camel Pose can be put toward more challenging poses, making Camel Pose a useful means of support and stability for your body and your yoga practice.

YOUR REACTION TO OTHERS TEACHES YOU ABOUT YOURSELF

What we often find problematic in others are the qualities and habits we dislike within ourselves. Witnessing a particular behavior in someone can hold a mirror up to our own behavior, and because we wish we didn't possess that habit or act in that particular way, we feel annoyed at the other person for revealing it to us. But if we shift our thinking about this issue, we can use our own reactions to others as a way to learn about ourselves. Notice your reactions to those around you today and ask yourself: *Where is this in me?* You may gain insights into yourself.

HONOR YOURSELF TODAY

Today, acknowledge your achievements and your creativity. Think about what you have said and what you have done that was positive and productive in the world. Look at who you are now and how you have grown and changed. With all this in mind, contemplate the complex and unique wonder that is you. Make the choice to fully embrace your body, your mind, and your heart right here and now. Congratulate yourself for all that you have done and been and for all that you will do and be. Think of today as a day of gratitude, by yourself and for yourself. Honor yourself today.

GROUND
YOURSELF

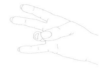

Prthivi Mudra (PRIT-ti-vee MOO-drah)
Earth Mudra

Sometimes, to ground ourselves, we need to find
a focus. Forming a mudra, or yogic hand gesture,
can offer us this focus. *Prthivi* is the Sanskrit word
for Earth. When we rest our hands palms up on our
thighs, and touch our ring fingers to our thumbs,
we create *Prthivi Mudra*, evoking the earth and our
connection to it. No matter what is happening in
our lives and in the world around us, we can use
Prthivi Mudra to calm ourselves, reminding us of
how the ground beneath us offers us support.

YOGA IS: A PRAYER OF GRATITUDE SPOKEN THROUGH YOUR BODY

Each yoga practice session is an honoring of your body articulated through movement and breath. You begin by sitting, eyes closed, palms together in prayer. You set your intention, and then start to move. As you move, you find strength and openness. Think of each pose as an offering that celebrates your embodied existence. Your practice becomes a gesture of thankfulness for what you have been given—a prayer of gratitude, spoken elegantly and reverently through your body.

WE DON'T NEED TO MAKE SOMEONE WRONG TO MAKE OURSELVES RIGHT

Sometimes to assert our identity in the world, we criticize someone else. On a certain level, this is natural—we learn through comparison and contrast, and we observe the behaviors of others to help develop a sense of ourselves. But if we fall into the habit of identifying ourselves by saying "I'm not like that," or "I don't do what she is doing," or "I would never say the things that he says," we are doing ourselves a disservice. Our lives are intertwined with the lives of those around us, but we are not defined by them. We can assert who we are without disparaging someone else. We can talk about what we value without declaring that someone with different values is wrong. The beauty of life is in its diversity: of looks, of opinions, of backgrounds, and of preferences. Try to assert who you are instead of who you are not, and support others in their different assertions of who they are. The world is richer for it.

YOGA IS: MOVEMENT

When we move on our yoga mats, we open our bodies and celebrate the fact that we are embodied beings. Within and without, we are pulsing with movement: the flow of our breath and our blood, the placing of our hands and feet on our mats, the arranging of our limbs, the shifting of our weight. Through our movement, we create connections in our bodies from top to bottom, front to back. Our movements may be strong and muscular, delicate and graceful, sinuous or abrupt. Our bodies are in a constant state of motion, and through our yoga practice, we begin to move in a more conscious, articulate way.

REVERSE YOUR PATTERNS
TO FIND EASE

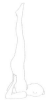

SHOULDER STAND POSE
SARVANGASANA (sar-VAN-GAH-sah-nah)

We spend most of our waking life sitting or standing. When we reverse gravity's effects by turning
upside down, we find ease from our usual patterns.
Sarvangasana, the Sanskrit word for Shoulder
Stand Pose, is a stable, grounded inversion that
requires a moderate degree of strength. Start by
lying on your back, facing the ceiling. Wiggle your
shoulder blades under your back for support, which
creates a lift for the neck so your vertebrae are not
pressing into the ground. Lift your pelvis and legs
into the air, and support your back with your hands.
Then relax, breathe, and enjoy the ease that comes
from reversing the force of gravity in your body.

THERE IS NO WRONG EMOTION

You are never wrong to feel a particular emotion. You feel whatever you feel. The question is: What will you do with what you are feeling? If you stay mired in an emotion that adversely affects you, such as jealousy or anger, you may need to work to change it. But this does not mean that you were wrong to feel it to begin with. So, first allow yourself to feel what you are feeling. Look at it; mentally poke at it. Remind yourself what the opposite of this emotion feels like, and see if it is possible to shift your experience to an emotion that benefits you when you feel ready to move on.

MAKE A DAILY
GRATITUDE LIST

Appreciate the richness of your life by weaving the feeling of gratitude into your entire day. When you wake up in the morning, make a mental list of five people or things for which you are grateful. Take a few minutes to think about each entry on your list. You might feel grateful toward a particular person or for a positive event that you experienced. You may feel good about one of your talents or accomplishments. You may simply feel thankful for the sun pouring in your window, or for your breakfast. This simple gratitude practice can set an appreciative tone for how you will move through the world today.

TURN DOING WHAT YOU LOVE INTO MEDITATION

When we want to relax or find ease, we often turn to meditation. But we can sometimes find a similarly meditative experience in doing a thing that we love. For some people, this could be walking or running, and for others it might be cooking, drawing, or engaging in any activity that offers us a sense of calm and focus. It often helps if the activity has a repetitive quality so it creates a meditative rhythm that lulls us. Today, decide to engage in an activity that you love as a form of meditation.

YOUR SPINE IS A BALANCE OF SUPPLENESS AND POWER

Your spine is a powerful network of bones that snakes its way from your pelvis up to your skull. Its curves support and distribute your weight. Your spine bends back and forth, side to side, and twists. Draw your attention to your spine right now. You may be sitting, standing, or lying down. Notice how your spine is shaped in its current position. Then, as you continue on with your day, notice the many different ways in which you move your spine. Imagine tracing each undulating line you form with your spine in every position you take. Each graceful curve is a balance of suppleness and power.

THE MYTH OF SHIVA NATARAJA AND THE SAGES IN THE FOREST

The sage Patanjali ventured into the forest, hoping to see the god Shiva Nataraja perform his exquisite Dance of Bliss. He encountered a Linga, a symbol of Shiva. It had been ornamented with pristine white blossoms. He thought that if he could offer the Linga more of these blossoms, Shiva might appear and reveal his dance, but he searched in vain. Exhausted, he curled up on the forest floor and slept. When he awoke, he was in the company of the sage Vyaghrapada, who had brought the white blossoms from his home in the treetops. Patanjali realized that he needed to offer gifts reflecting his own origins and journey, rather than seeking to provide gifts that others had offered. And so he gathered seeds from the forest floor. When the two sages brought their gifts together before the Linga, it transformed into Shiva Nataraja, who performed his beautiful Dance of Bliss. Like Patanjali, we need to recognize that our own gifts are what we can best offer to the world, and that this will give us access to beauty.

BREATHE INTO YOUR FEET TO GROUND AND NOURISH YOURSELF

When we breathe, we draw oxygen into our cells. We nourish our entire body, all the way down to our feet. In this way, with each breath, we ground ourselves to the earth. Remember this as you move through your day today. Periodically stop and take a deep inhale. Invite the breath to move all the way through your body and down into the soles of your feet to connect with the ground beneath you. Remind yourself that your breath affects your entire body, and that each time you inhale, you steady and nourish yourself.

THE HEAT OF YOUR YOGA PRACTICE WILL TRANSFORM YOU

In your yoga practice, you build heat. Heat causes transformation. Think of the alchemy of mixing and warming ingredients to cook a meal. When you move your body into poses on your mat, you create an internal heat that equally cooks and transforms you. Since you are a being made of an intertwined body, mind, and heart; the warmth you build in your body transforms your entire physical, mental, and spiritual self. The Sanskrit word *tapas* (TAH-pahs) means heat, energy, and the discipline of your practice. Your yoga will transform you through your *tapas*, through the heat of your practice.

THERE IS A TIME TO SPEAK AND A TIME TO LISTEN

While it is often important to make our voices heard, there are also times when it is more important to listen. When we listen to the ideas and values of others, we learn more about the world, expanding our own ideas in the process. Then, when it is our turn to speak, we do so from a thoughtful, well-informed place. We benefit when we find a balance between listening to other people's ideas and articulating our own. Notice today if you can find a balance between listening to others and articulating your own thoughts. See if you can represent who you are and what you care about while respecting others' ideas and values.

ACCESSING
PEACE

Take a moment today to close your eyes and think
of something that gives you a sense of deep peace
and equilibrium. Is it a place such as the ocean or
a mountaintop? Is it a specific song that calms and
quiets you? Or is it a moment, like sitting quietly
with a cup of tea? Connect with one thing that
evokes the power of peace for you. This thing is
your gateway to a peaceful state. Whenever you
need peace, reconnect with it. Peace will always
be available to you by just closing your eyes.

THE DIFFERENCE BETWEEN
HABIT AND RITUAL

Though habit and ritual are sometimes thought to be the same, there is a difference between them. A habit is an action or a behavior that we repeat, often mechanically, out of convenience or comfort. A ritual, on the other hand, is an action that we consciously choose to repeat with awareness and intentionality. While habits are rote, rituals are mindful; they actually create and hold meaning. Today, begin to develop your awareness of your habits so you can decide whether they serve you. Retain them if they do and discard them if they don't. Also, begin to consider how you can establish rituals that consciously create meaning in your life. In doing so, you honor what is significant, beautiful, and worthy of your attention.

OPEN YOUR
HEART

Hridaya Mudra (hri-dah-yah MOO-drah)
Mudra of the Heart

When we speak of opening our hearts, we are talking about the experience of finding spaciousness and beauty within ourselves. Curl your index finger to touch the base of your thumb, then touch the tip of your thumb to the tips of your middle and ring fingers, and extend your pinkie. This is the mudra, or hand gesture, of *hridaya*, the Sanskrit word for heart. Dense and complex, yet elegantly opening, *Hridaya Mudra* reminds us to always open to the graceful complexity that resides within our hearts.

SELF-ACCEPTANCE SETS US FREE

When we accept ourselves and our life circumstances, we are better able to move forward.
When we dwell on what we could have done, how
we could be if we were not who we are, or what we
don't like about ourselves, we imprison ourselves in
a cage of regret and useless self-criticism. Acceptance begins with acknowledgment: this is who we
are, this is what we have done, this is the way things
are, like it or not. Try accepting these realities, and
then working with them. Personal progress begins
with self-acceptance. And self-acceptance will set
us free.

SHED AN OLD HABIT TO CREATE A NEW ONE

Sometimes we realize that a particular habit of ours no longer serves our best interests. At some point, it may have been the best way of addressing a set of circumstances in our life, but over time, it has lost its effectiveness. It has become rote behavior, an automatic response to a given situation. Do you remember that article of clothing you loved to wear when you were little? It suited you then, but it doesn't now. Think of your habits like clothing you wear until it no longer fits you. Today, notice your habitual behavior. Ask yourself: *Does this habit serve me today?* And if it doesn't, shed it in favor of a new behavior.

CULTIVATE YOUR INNER POWER

We are powerful. The power of our bodies enables us to move on our mats, to dance, to run, to celebrate our embodied experience. The power of our minds is equally important, generating creativity, ingenuity, insight, and wisdom. The power of our hearts enables us to give and receive love, to care for others and practice empathy in the world. The question is: How will you use your power? Generally, the more empowered we feel, the more likely we are to use our power toward positive ends. Today, take note of some way you are powerful. Then use that power to offer others an experience of their empowerment, too.

ENGAGE WITH LIFE

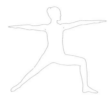

WARRIOR II POSE
VIRABHADRASANA II (VI-rah-bah-DRA-sah-nah)

How fully are you living your life? *Virabhadrasana II* is the Sanskrit name for Warrior II Pose, often called *Vira II*. The word *vira* means hero or warrior, or to be fully engaged with life. When you stand in *Vira II*—front leg in a lunge, back leg extended and foot anchored to the ground, arms outstretched over your legs—each of your limbs is actively engaged and your body is engaged and expansive. To be *vira* means to open yourself to what life offers, embracing all of its challenges and triumphs. To be *vira* is to say yes to life in all of its complexity. To be *vira* means to have the courage and tenacity to step forward into your day with a heroic and ferocious love of life.

DEALING WITH CHANGE

How do you deal with change? Do you resist or do you accept? Do you fight it or do you adapt and move forward? There is a time to let things dissolve and a time to re-form. This ebb and flow is the nature of all things, so the best we can do is adapt to this process in our lives, releasing the past, aligning with the present, and moving forward into the future. Like a plant that flowers, dies, and then feeds the soil for a new plant to grow, we exist in a perpetual cycle of change. The more we accept this, the more we grow.

FINDING WONDER IN YOUR BODY'S SURFACE

Your skin is the largest organ of your body. It has the most surface area, the greatest amount of exposure of any of your organs to the outside world, and it presents you with constant information about the temperature, texture, and overall nature of your surroundings. Take a moment today to direct your attention to everything that is in contact with your skin. Notice the textures and friction of your clothing. Notice any other materials with which your skin is in contact: a seat, the floor, the air. Take note of the temperature and the movement of the air and what that feels like. Allow yourself to find wonder in the complex sensations experienced by your body's surface.

I INVITE BEAUTY, ABUNDANCE, AND GOOD FORTUNE INTO MY LIFE

Om Shrim Maha Lakshmyai Namaha
(ohm shreem mah-hah lah-kshmyai nah-mah-ha)

This mantra invokes Lakshmi, goddess of beauty, abundance, and good fortune. Lakshmi loves light. To invite her into your home, place a candle or light in the window, and chant to her. *Om* evokes everything that exists. *Shrim* is a syllable associated with Lakshmi, containing her potency. *Maha* means great. *Lakshmyai* is the way we chant her name in the mantra. *Namaha* means that we bow down, we honor. When we chant *Om Shrim Maha Lakshmyai Namaha*, we invite beauty, prosperity, and good fortune into our lives.

DON'T BE AFRAID TO
BE YOURSELF

You may hold different ideas and have different habits from the people around you. You may look different or may choose to present yourself differently. Your differences are your uniqueness, and in your uniqueness resides your creativity, so treasure it. Know that what you bring to the table is as good and as interesting as what anyone else brings, and that your distinctive point of view matters. Be authentically you and influence the world with your originality and lack of fear about being exceptional. Don't be afraid to be yourself.

DAYDREAM TO TAP INTO YOUR CREATIVE LIFE

Creativity takes a balance of disciplined work and unstructured time to let your mind wander. When you daydream, you tap into your creative self: your unarticulated thoughts, your questions about the world, and your ability to make surprising associations. Daydreaming is a valuable part of the creative process. Take a few minutes today and let your mind drift. Watch where it goes and notice what thoughts and ideas arise. Scribble down some notes, doodle, or make a voice memo. Like sleeping dreams, daydreams can be nonsensical and odd, but these are the sources from which creativity and original thought tend to come. Give yourself time to daydream a little bit every day.

MEDITATION IS WATCHING YOUR THOUGHTS

Sometimes meditation can be as simple as observing your thoughts to notice what you are thinking about. This process helps you discover your thought patterns. Becoming familiar with these patterns is empowering, offering you a greater awareness of your mental state so you are not merely subject to the intensity of your thoughts and emotions. Watching your thoughts offers you the space to inwardly sit back and observe the wonder of your own mind. As a thought pattern arises, you can say to yourself, *Oh, here this is again*, and by acknowledging it, release it. You can sit in meditation, watching your thoughts as if you were sitting in a field, watching clouds go by: observant, calm, and peaceful.

SPEAK TO YOURSELF WITH LOVE

Today, notice your self-talk, meaning how you talk to yourself about yourself. Take note of whether you congratulate yourself for your successes or denigrate yourself when you don't achieve your goals. Do you dwell on what you like about yourself in a way that encourages you? Or are you excessively self-critical? Often, what we articulate either out loud or in the privacy of our own minds and hearts sets the stage for the reality that we will live. Our thoughts to ourselves about ourselves can either elevate or limit us. Today, if you notice yourself mentally lodged in a place of self-criticism or harsh self-talk, actively shift this behavior by refocusing on your positive qualities, choosing to speak to yourself with love.

YOU ARE THE LOTUS BLOSSOM

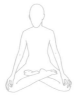

LOTUS POSE
PADMASANA (pahd-MAH-sah-nah)

Rooted in the earth, the lotus rises up through the water to blossom in the sunlight. Similarly, we are at our best when we are grounded in who we are, always moving forward, and opening up expansively to embrace life. When we bend our knees to tuck our feet onto our upper thighs in *Padmasana*, the Sanskrit word for Lotus Pose, we form the shape of a lotus with our lower bodies. *Padmasana* is deeply grounding, which is why it is used for meditation. The next time you sit for meditation, take *Padmasana* or its simpler cross-legged version, close your eyes, and envision yourself rooted in the earth, rising upward like the stem, and unfolding like lotus petals in the sun to exuberantly receive life.

OFFER COMPASSION TO CREATE A BETTER WORLD

When we are more compassionate toward others, we help create a better world. Even the smallest gesture of compassion has the potential to ripple outward. Think of how it feels when someone offers you kindness when you are having a tough day. That person's gesture shifts your perception of your situation in that particular moment, reminding you that you matter and that people care. It makes you more likely to offer a similar kindness to another person. So today, offer kindness and compassion to someone you encounter, and know that you are helping to create a better world.

THE WISDOM OF MULTIPLE PERSPECTIVES

The way we look at a situation is influenced by our personal histories and life experiences. When we recognize how our experiences have shaped our perspective, we begin to understand that our opinions and values are distinctly our own: no one shares our exact point of view because no one has lived our exact personal history. We begin to see that our point of view is unique. This realization enables us to recognize that there are as many unique points of view as there are people in the world, and that all have validity. Yoga teaches us that we are wiser when we listen to and learn from a diversity of perspectives.

THE MYTH OF KRISHNA IN THE MARKETPLACE

One day, when Krishna was a baby, his mother, Yashoda, brought him with her to the market-place and placed him underneath her butter cart to keep him safe while she conducted business. Baby Krishna, who adored his mother and always wanted to be hugged and held by her, cried to get her attention. But Yashoda, who was busy with her marketing, ignored his cries, assuming that he would eventually stop demanding her attention and quiet down. Eventually, Krishna couldn't stand being ignored any longer. Propelled by love, he used all of his divine power to overturn the heavy butter cart. The pots cracked, spilling milk and butter all over the ground. Yashoda rushed to pick up Krishna, worried that he had been injured in the accident. She had no idea that her small but powerful baby had overturned the entire cart. This myth shows us that love's power can surprise us in the most amazing ways.

THE EXPERIENCE
OF FULLNESS

What does fullness feel like to you? To some people it feels like contentment or satisfaction. To others, fullness evokes a state of being on the verge of overflowing with love. Fullness can feel like satisfaction, a deep sense of calm, or an expansive sense of joy. Fullness may feel like completion—as if there is nothing you need to change. The experience of fullness cannot be completely described. When your heart is so rich with feeling that you have no words, that is fullness.

LEARNING TO LISTEN TO OTHERS

Listening can be one of the most difficult skills to master. We are sometimes so eager to express ourselves, to share our experiences and to be understood, that we neglect the equally important part of communication—listening. Without listening, we are trapped in our own limited ways of thinking and points of view. We don't stop advocating our own ideas long enough to recognize that there is a world of ideas out there to which we have access. Listening allows us to expand our minds and our imaginations. Listening is the key to learning and growing as human beings. Try to speak less today. Pause and listen to what is being said.

YOGA IS: WISDOM

Yoga is much more than the physical movement of our bodies on yoga mats. Yoga also offers us insights into our motivations, our desires, and the ways in which we think and feel about ourselves. We can broaden our experience of yoga by exploring yoga philosophy and mythology. This approach is called *Jnana* (NYAH-nah) *Yoga*. The Sanskrit word *jnana* means wisdom, and *Jnana Yoga* means the yoga of wisdom. In our lives as yoga practitioners, we can cultivate an intelligence of both our bodies and our minds. Wisdom can be found in every corner of yoga, whether we are moving on our mats, meditating on a cushion, or reading ancient texts. Yoga is wisdom.

FIND GRACE WITHIN POWER

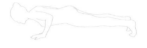

FOUR LIMBED STAFF POSE
CHATURANGA DANDASANA (chaht-too-RAN-gah dahn-DAH-sah-nah)

Can you combine strength with ease? One of the most difficult yoga poses to hold, *Chaturanga Dandasana*, the Sanskrit name for Four Limbed Staff Pose, looks like the lowered-down part of a push-up, and it entails determination and endurance. To stay in the pose, engage your abdominal muscles and extend forward through the top of your head and back through your heels. In Sanskrit, *chatur* means four, and *anga* means limbs. In this pose, your body is the *danda*—the Sanskrit word for staff—that is supported by your four limbs, calling upon all of your patience and graceful power to hover just inches above the ground.

WHEN IT'S RIGHT
TO BE FIERCE

Ferocity can be a positive quality when directed in the proper way. When we have to defend someone who has been wronged, ferocity can be the appropriate reaction or attitude. To be fierce can mean speaking in a fiery, determined, passionate way about what we care about and pledging to support what we believe in. Think of causes that you care about, people who need to be defended, standing up for your rights or for the rights of others. Embrace ferocity when the moment for it arises.

THE IMPORTANCE OF GIVING BACK

Consider how you can be generous with those who are generous with you. And consider how you can be generous to the world, which has given you so much. Think of the people who have helped you in your life. When you look at what they have given you, imagine how you could give back to them. Also imagine what you could give to others, following the lead of those who have given so much to you. When you give to those who need help as well as to those who have helped you, you step into a cycle of generosity and giving. You begin to participate more deeply in the generative flow of the universe.

ACCEPTING WHAT WE DON'T UNDERSTAND

Most of our life is a mystery. We will never know why certain things happen, exactly how our bodies work, or why we are here. We can spend a lifetime learning about the universe and still not understand how it functions. By accepting and appreciating that we are lifelong learners, we can enjoy our lives more fully. We are part of an enormous tapestry, of which we cannot see the beginning or end. We know only our particular view from our particular place. When we embrace living in this state of mystery, we can begin to find the beauty in it.

MEDITATE ON TASTE
AND SMELL

Yoga offers us a heightened awareness of the world. Along with a greater understanding of how our bodies move comes a similar awareness of our bodies' other physical functions. Today, direct this awareness to your senses of taste and smell. At each meal, slow down, think of what you are about to put into your body, and focus on smell, texture, and taste as you prepare and eat your food. Don't read, flip through your phone, use your computer, or watch TV. Simply explore the rich sensory experience of eating meditatively. Give as much reverence to your meals as you would your yoga practice, and see how it shifts your daily experience.

YOGA WILL WAKE YOU UP

When you start a yoga practice, you may notice that your body begins to change: your muscles feel more open and less constricted, you feel more physically at ease, and your skin may even feel vibrant. You may begin to notice a parallel set of experiences happening in your attitude and disposition: your mind feels more energized and creative, and your heart feels more generous and receptive. It is as if you have been roused from slumber. Yoga will wake you up.

THE MYTH OF KALI'S WILD DANCE

The demon Raktabija had been terrorizing the world, and none of the gods could stop him, so they called to the ferocious goddess Kali for help. Kali unleashed her ferocity to defeat Raktabija, and began triumphantly dancing on the battlefield. The gods watched, alarmed, as her dancing became increasingly frenzied and out of control. While they had needed Kali's ferocity to conquer the demon, they now needed her to calm down. They called to Kali's beloved, Shiva, god of dissolution, to help. Shiva arrived and stretched out on the battlefield, emanating stillness. Lost in her ecstatic dance, Kali began to trample Shiva, but as she felt his body beneath her feet, her movements slowed until she was swaying back and forth blissfully on top of him. Shiva's stillness had soothed Kali's frenzy, and balance was restored to the world. Like Kali, we can use our strengths for good, but, in excess, they may draw us out of alignment. Today, how can you use your strengths to take action in the world and still maintain your equilibrium?

YOUR BREATH IS A RIVER

Your breath is like a body of water, sometimes shallow, other times deep, always rising and falling. You breathe air into your lungs, but the energy of the breath travels everywhere in your body, as oxygen is invited into all of your cells. When you finish reading this paragraph, close your eyes and inhale. Imagine the breath, like a river, moving through your body and extending through smaller tributaries into your limbs, feet, and hands. Your body becomes a landscape, nourished by the ebb and flow of your breath.

YOGA IS:
ASANA

The Sanskrit word *asana* (AH-sah-nah) means
a seat or a pose, which is why you sometimes hear
the physical practice of yoga referred to as *Yoga
Asana*. You also see and hear the word *asana* at the
end of yoga pose names written in Sanskrit—for
example, *Dandasana* (dan-DAH-sah-nah), which is
also known as Staff Pose (*danda* means staff). Each
asana invites you to take a specific "seat" in order
to answer a question or solve a problem with your
body: *How do I experience myself in Triangle Pose
as opposed to Handstand? How does my breathing change from pose to pose? What can I learn
about myself through movement and breath? What
do I feel within my body in each asana?* When you
perform any *asana*, you take a particular seat
of inquiry. Through this process, you learn about
yourself. Your body becomes aware, articulate,
and intelligent. *Yoga Asana* cultivates an intelligence of the body.

CHOOSE YOUR WORDS WITH PRECISION

Today, when you find yourself in conversation, take a pause before speaking. In that suspended moment, clearly identify what you want to express. Ask yourself: *Is what I truly want to say about to emerge from my mouth?* Then, thoughtfully choose the words that will most accurately convey what you want to say. There is a beautiful integrity to choosing your words with precision and intention. Your mouth is halfway between your mind and your heart. Let these two centers of intelligence converge to create more meaningful self-expression.

CONNECT WITH NATURE TO CONNECT WITH YOURSELF

Connecting with nature helps us connect with our bodies and with the world around us. Whether we live in the country or the city, there is always a way to connect with nature. If you can go to the woods, the ocean, or a park, place your bare feet on the earth as often as possible. Pay special attention to trees, plants, or even cut flowers or potted plants in your home. Notice the beauty and complexity of their surfaces, and imagine the structures beneath their surfaces that cause growth, change, and transformation. In this way, these other natural beings are like us. Connecting with nature reminds us that we are part of nature, and that to appreciate ourselves, we must appreciate that connection.

MAKE AN OFFERING TO THE WORLD

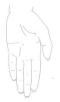

Varada Mudra (vah-rah-dah MOO-drah)
Mudra of Offering

What can you contribute to the world? How can you use your talents and gifts to give to the people around you? *Varada Mudra* is the hand gesture of offering, giving, and generosity. Usually done by placing the left hand palm up on the left knee, *Varada Mudra* signifies our making an offering. The offering can be of our thoughts, of our minds, or of our intentions. *Varada Mudra* can signify the literal giving of a gift, and it can also be a gesture of sweetness and abundance—a type of blessing. Any mudra is an invitation to yourself, so *Varada Mudra* invites you to offer abundance and support to yourself as well as to those around you.

SURRENDER TO MOVE FORWARD

Surrendering doesn't mean giving up your authority; it means accepting what is unchangeable instead of fighting a battle that you cannot win. Surrendering involves knowing the difference between what you are capable of changing and what you are not capable of changing, then figuring out how to come to terms with that reality. When you feel as if you are banging your head against an unmovable wall, that is a good time to surrender. Just as there is a give and take to everything in life, there are times when all the pushing in the world won't get you what you want. Let go, releasing your old thinking in order to re-form a relationship that will work with you, not against you.

WHAT WE WANT AND WHAT WE NEED

What is the difference between our wants and our needs? Our needs—such as food, health, and shelter—are necessary to our survival. Our wants, while not necessary, can still meaningfully enhance our lives. To lead healthy lives, we must first distinguish our needs from our wants. Ask yourself: *What is essential to my well-being?* Once we have addressed our needs, we can then ask ourselves: *Which of my wants will positively affect my life? Which will bring me healthiness, happiness, stability, and peace of mind?* In this manner, we can embrace the pleasure of our wants in a healthy, joyful, and meaningful way.

OPEN AND RECEIVE THE WORLD

Through a physical yoga practice, we cultivate openness in our bodies. It is equally important to cultivate openness in our minds and our hearts. But how do we create this openness off the mat? To open is to soften the barriers we put up between ourselves and the world. Opening can be a physical sensation, like the relaxing of muscles or the loosening of a tight jaw. Opening can be the easing of our defenses—enabling us, for example, to hear what others have to say even when it is unfamiliar or in disagreement with what we think and believe. Opening invites us to connect more deeply with the world around us. When we open to receive the world, we are received by the world.

SHAPE
YOUR DAY

Choose one word that symbolizes the experience you wish to have today. The word could be energy, ease, hope, curiosity, peace, or whatever quality or state of mind inspires and motivates you. Say the word out loud so it resonates in your body. Write it down so it feels like a commitment. This is your intention, or the way in which you want to move through your life today. An intention, like an anchor, keeps you steady and focused. Throughout your day, return to this word. Recommit to it. Your intention has the power to shape your day.

STAY GROUNDED
WHILE GROWING

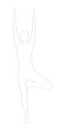

TREE POSE
VRKSASANA (vri-KSHA-sah-nah)

Can you be grounded and inspired at the same time? Can you stay centered while dreaming of greatness? *Vrksasana* is the Sanskrit name for Tree Pose. In *Vrksasana,* you plant one foot sturdily on the ground as if putting down roots, and brace your other foot against your standing leg. Then you reach your arms up toward the sky like branches. On and off the mat, you can remain grounded in who you are while continuing to grow and change. First, establish your foundation: *This is who I am.* Next, expand into your potential: *This is who I want to be.* Look beyond the treetops of everything you know about yourself, and dream.

ARRIVE AT YOUR MAT IN A WAY THAT HONORS YOUR YOGA PRACTICE

How we present ourselves to the world—in a social interaction or a work environment, for example—expresses something about our attitudes toward the people in our lives and the settings we inhabit. Similarly, how we present ourselves on our yoga mat expresses something about our attitudes toward ourselves and our practice. Honor your practice by arriving with an attitude that expresses the reverence you feel for it: for example, arranging your mat carefully on the floor, then moving slowly and intentionally as you place your body on your mat, appreciating the rituals that set the stage for your practice session. In doing so, you honor yoga. You honor yourself.

WE ARE ONE AND WE ARE MANY

Each of us is a unique individual. Each of us has particular tastes, preferences, and talents. Each of us has our own personal way of being in the world. But folded into our individual selves are many different selves, each one formed from the diversity of our experiences and the cultivation, over time, of our tastes and sensibilities. We are made up of many and yet we are one. When we feel powerless or blocked, this is what we need to remember: We are infinite. We hold limitless possibility. We are one and we are many.

I BOW DOWN TO THE UNIVERSAL POWER OF TRANSFORMATION

Om Gam Ganapataye Namaha
(ohm gahm gah-nah-pat-tah-ye nah-mah-ha)

Change. Newness. Transformation. When we chant to yoga mythology's elephant-headed god Ganesha, as we do with this mantra, we are invoking our powers of transformation, we are inviting a shift where one is needed in our lives, and we are embracing the bittersweetness of change. *Om* evokes everything that exists. *Gam* is Ganesha's "seed syllable," meaning it contains his power in the way that an acorn contains an oak tree. *Ganapataye* is how we sing his name in the mantra, and *Namaha* means that we bow down, we honor. When we chant *Om Gam Ganapataye Namaha*, we call to our deepest abilities to create change, to step into a new place in our lives, and to do so with decisiveness and grace.

THE IMPORTANCE OF BEING BY YOURSELF

Schedule a day this week when you can reserve some time to enjoy your own company. Dedicate this time to exploring the mix of thoughts, ideas, and dreams that make you who you are. While there is a clear benefit to bouncing your ideas off others and sharing experiences, balancing your public self with your private self can nurture and affirm your personal value. You become more settled in yourself and more certain in how you wish to present yourself in the world. Instead of surrounding yourself with people, for just a few hours this week, immerse yourself in you.

FOCUS YOUR VISION TO FOCUS YOUR LIFE

In yoga, the Sanskrit word *drshti* (DRISH-tee) can mean seeing, point of view, or inner vision. It can also refer to the act of gazing at a focal point. Practicing *drshti* can be as simple as staring at the flickering flame of a candle during meditation, or choosing a spot on the wall to look at to help maintain our balance in a yoga pose. To focus means to steady ourselves, to direct our attention, to concentrate. To do this, we have to reduce the distractions that surround us. Through *drshti*, we temporarily narrow the scope of our vision, so that we can dive more deeply into one specific place or state of mind. We temporarily put on blinders so we can have a deep experience of one thing rather than a broad experience of many things. In this way, we begin to direct not just our attention but also our lives.

FINDING TRANQUILITY WHEREVER WE ARE

The next time you find yourself in the middle of a noisy, jostling crowd, or stuck in traffic, or confronted by confusion or disorder, take a deep breath. Feel the breath move all the way down from your chest, belly, and hips, through your legs and feet, and into the ground. No matter where you are or what your circumstances may be, you can always create an experience of tranquility. Tranquility is an inner state, not an external event or destination. When we focus on the breath and on the inner body, we remind ourselves of the existence of our internal world where tranquility resides—a personal space of quiet and calm to which we can return when needed.

GROUND YOURSELF THROUGH MEDITATION

Meditation is a practice that can clear your mind or focus it. It can bring you energy or a feeling of ease, and it can ground you, meaning that it can settle your body, heart, and mind. The next time you feel scattered or uncertain, try this grounding meditation. Begin by slowing down. Take a seat if you can, or try it standing up. Close your eyes. Pay attention to the rise and fall of your breath inside your body. Then, with each inhale, notice how it feels to be connected to the surface on which you are sitting or standing. Notice how the chair supports your weight, or, if you're standing, how the floor supports your feet. Then imagine connecting even further into the ground, as if you were extending roots down into the earth beneath you. With every breath, ground yourself more and more deeply.

BE LIKE
WATER

When we really want something, we can be forceful.
We assert and we push. Sometimes forcefulness
is what the situation calls for. Other times, it doesn't
work. Sometimes, to get what we want, we need to
yield, to soften, so that we can navigate what the
world is offering us. Think of how water wears down
the surface of rocks and the edges of glass, pol-
ishing their sharp, gritty surfaces into smoothly
sculpted objects. Today, when pushing doesn't work,
try mentally stepping back and fluidly receiving
what you are experiencing. Witness how your softness can be a source of strength.

HOLDING OURSELVES
WITH LOVE

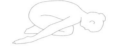

CHILD'S POSE
BALASANA (BAH-LA-sah-nah)

Can you treat yourself with love? Can you hold
yourself in the same gentle way you would a child
or a loved one? *Balasana* is the Sanskrit name for
Child's Pose. When we gently fold forward into
Balasana, we feel held, safe, nurtured. Our pulse
quiets and we begin to relax. Our ability to hold
and nurture others is infinitely greater when we
learn to hold and nurture ourselves. In *Balasana*,
we hold ourselves lightly but sweetly, curled in
toward our own center. Caring for others begins
with self-care.

GENERATE
KINDNESS

As you move through your day today, acknowledge the people you meet, offering them basic and polite respect. Sometimes simply saying hello or thank you makes a far greater difference to that person than you might imagine. We never know what is happening in another person's life, and the smallest gesture can make others feel that they are not invisible, that they are worthy of acknowledgment, that they matter. And this is a great gift to give. Sometimes you will receive the same type of respect that you have offered, and other times you will not. It doesn't matter, because the point is not about reciprocity. The point is about generating thoughtfulness and kindness in the world. Try it for a day, not looking for outside affirmation, but looking within yourself, feeling good about who you are in the world and that you have made it a kinder place in which to live.

LET THE WORLD
SING TO YOU

Wherever you are right now, open your senses. What
are you seeing all around you at this moment?
What are you hearing, from the sound of your breath
to the most distant sounds? Where are you seated,
and what are the bodily sensations created by the
textures of your surroundings? What smells
register strongly and faintly? The world can be an
operatic experience—an artwork made of layers
of cascading sensory information—if you let it. You
simply have to pay attention. Let the world sing
to you through all of your senses.

HONOR EACH DAY
OF YOUR LIFE

Treat each morning as a new beginning—a vast landscape of opportunity inviting you to step in and to
engage. Whether your day is free or scheduled from
beginning to end, your experience of it is your creative choice. Each day has the potential for beauty
and satisfaction if you look for them and are open
to receiving them. As you move through your day
today, notice how you are in a state of creative possibility. Honor what you make out of your choices.
Choose to embrace gratitude for each opportunity
to co-create with everything around you.

A MYTH OF BRAHMA
AND GANESHA

The sweet elephant-headed god Ganesha was wandering along a shady path of the forest. As he moved between the trees, he was so distracted by the warmth, the jasmine-scented air, and the ripe fruit on the trees that he stopped paying attention to the path. He turned a corner and collided with the great creator god Brahma, who was knocked into the dust. Irate at the younger god's care-lessness, Brahma opened his mouth to curse him, but just as he began to speak, Ganesha smiled apologetically and began to dance. His enormous body caused the earth to quiver and the trees to rain down fruit and blossoms. Seeing this, Brahma decided to release his anger, and forgave Ganesha for his mistake. Like Brahma, we can't choose what happens to us, but we can change how we choose to receive our experience.

YOU ARE MORE THAN YOUR BODY

In addition to that which makes up our body—sinew, bone, muscle, and fiber—there is within us what we call spirit. Spirit does not have a shape or form. It cannot be located in a photograph or touched with our fingers. Rather, it is a felt thing, an intuited thing, residing in our cells but not limited to the confines of our bodies. Unlike our bodies, which are bound by the limits of a physical existence, our spirits are limitless. Today, notice what you intuit and sense. Notice what you find yourself dreaming about or imagining. These are experiences of spirit. Honor them as you honor your bodily experiences of taste and touch, sight and smell. Embrace your spiritual self.

CULTIVATE ATTENTIVENESS TO EXPERIENCE WONDER

Today, create an opportunity to experience wonder. Seek out and focus on something very small, like a leaf or a flower petal. Take in its appearance, examining its shape, its color, its veins. Feel its texture and listen to the sound it makes as you move it between your fingertips. Notice if it has a smell. When you draw your attention to something this small in an extremely focused way, you are creating an opportunity to experience wonder. And if this small object can contain such richness, imagine the vast richness contained by the world. Invite yourself to be attentive to each tiny detail of the world in its complexity. Cultivating attentiveness offers us the experience of wonder.

YOGA IS: CONNECTION

The Sanskrit root of the word yoga is *yuj* (yoodge), which means to connect or to create connection. When we move on our mats, shifting our limbs, our muscles, our tissues, and our bones, we create positive, aligned connection within our bodies. When our bodies are physically aligned, our minds can more readily find an equivalent alignment, and our hearts can then share this sense of ease. Our physical, mental, and emotional selves enter into a more meaningful conversation with each other. Yoga offers the connection of our bodies to our minds and to our hearts.

THE DANCE OF LIFE

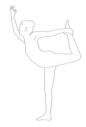

LORD OF THE DANCE POSE
NATARAJASANA (nah-tah-RAH-JAH-sah-nah)

Natarajasana is the Sanskrit name for Lord of the Dance Pose, or Dancer's Pose as it is also known. *Nata* means dancer and *raja* means lord or king. In yoga mythology, the powerful Hindu deity Shiva is called Nataraja when he dances. His dance demonstrates the cycle of life in all its beauty, challenges, and mystery. Balancing on one leg, reach back to hold your other bent leg in the air. *Natarajasana* reflects the passionate dance that is life. It reminds us that we are always dancing, always engaged in life's challenges. And it invites us to dance the challenges and beauty of our lives as meaningfully as possible.

YOGA IS: A COMMITMENT TO YOURSELF

When you choose to begin a yoga practice, you are engaging in a process of interweaving your body, your mind, and your heart. Sustaining that practice is a true commitment to yourself, but it is often a challenge. So how do you do it? To knit together your body, heart, and mind, you must first deepen your awareness of their connectivity. Notice how when you move your body on your mat, your mind may relax, and your heart opens. When you focus on this constant interplay, the three support each other and your commitment to yourself deepens.

PRACTICE GENEROSITY TO CREATE ABUNDANCE IN THE WORLD

What does it mean to practice generosity? There is a generosity of spirit, of body, and of material needs. Generosity can be about listening: being patient with a child or with a person who needs someone to talk to. Practicing generosity can be having tolerance for people's foibles and accepting their quirks and habits. Generosity can be about donating money or material goods to someone in need. Generosity is about giving of yourself in any number of ways, depending on what the situation necessitates, from listening to helping out. And if you are being truly generous, you are doing it without expectation of it being repaid. You do it to do it. Being generous to others brings abundance into their lives and into yours. You can generate more abundance in the world by practicing generosity.

MEDITATE ON THE SOUNDS AROUND YOU

Sometimes people think of meditation as a turning away from the world. But we are embodied beings who live in the world, so it is possible to embrace the world as a way of meditating. Close your eyes. Expand your awareness to notice what you hear around you: the sounds in the room, outside the room, then even farther, listening for the most distant sound you can hear. Instead of trying to ignore voices and ambient noise, invite them all in as part of the fabric of your meditation. Stay in this state of expansive awareness, allowing the world around you to contribute to your meditation practice. When you are ready, draw your attention back to your body, to your breath, and open your eyes.

YOU HAVE
PRESENCE

Take a seat, and notice how your body connects to the surface on which you are sitting. Then shift your attention to the places where your skin touches the air. Think to yourself: *This is where my body meets the world*. A thin layer of skin is all that separates your body from all that is not your body. And yet the energy of your body extends far beyond the parameters of your body. People sense you. People see and hear you. When you feel isolated or disconnected from the world, when you feel that your ideas and opinions are not being heard, stop for a moment. Take the time to notice this deep connectivity with the world around you. Remember that your body extends out into the world farther than you can imagine. You matter. You make an impact. You have presence.

THE MYTH OF MATSYENDRA

One day, the goddess Parvati said to her beloved husband, "Shiva, tell me the secrets of the universe." The great god Shiva, entranced by his wife's beauty and wisdom, agreed to do so, saying, "We must go to a place where no one can hear us." So they plunged into the ocean and swam down to its dark, rocky floor. Once there, Shiva began to speak. The secrets of the universe tumbled from his lips into her ear. When he finished, they detected a movement next to them. What they had thought was a rock was actually an enormous barnacle-covered fish. The fish began to speak: "Shiva, I have waited for thousands of years to know your secrets and I thank you." Shiva blessed him, saying, "Since you now know the secrets of the universe, I declare you to be a great sage named Matsyendra, Lord of the Fishes." Matsyendra then emerged from the ocean and began to teach. The myth of Matsyendra teaches us that practicing patience, dedication, and tenacity may lead to greatness.

REVERENCE OFFERS US THE EXPERIENCE OF GRATITUDE

To revere means to honor, respect, and venerate. To practice reverence, begin to soften and take in your surroundings. Notice the beauty of the details. Listen to people attentively, appreciating their thoughts and ideas. When we offer reverence, we experience gratitude, a deep experience of appreciation and thankfulness, because gratitude thrives on attentiveness and respect. Sometimes it is not until we act with reverence toward something that we are able to perceive its true beauty. Our reverence opens our eyes. Try it. Move through your day with reverence for yourself, the objects around you, and the people you meet, and notice how this affects you. Through reverence, we experience gratitude in our lives.

YOU ARE CONNECTED
TO THE UNIVERSE

Cin Mudra (chin MOO-drah)
Mudra of Consciousness

Arrange your hands in *Cin Mudra*, a hand gesture that signifies connection. *Cin* refers to consciousness. In *Cin Mudra*, your thumbs represent universal consciousness and your index fingers represent individual consciousness. By connecting your index fingers to your thumbs, you are connecting your individual consciousness to the greater universal consciousness. Your hands are symbolically mirroring that greater reality and inviting you to participate more deeply in this reality. By bringing the fingers together in *Cin Mudra*, you connect to everything that exists.

FOCUS ON THE BREATH TO EXPERIENCE THE MIRACULOUS

Inhale deeply. Notice how your breath fills your body, expanding your lungs and upper body. Exhale fully, allowing your body to relax and release. Continue breathing in this way, and as you do so, bring your attention back to this rise and fall, again and again. When other thoughts enter your mind, exhale them away, and invite yourself back to focus on the movement of the breath. Breathing is an involuntary reflex, rarely requiring our thought or attention. But when we choose to focus on it, it is transformed from a seemingly simple process to one that is rich and complex. Our bodies are miraculous.

BE FIERY WHEN
NEEDED

We often seek out yoga to find calm in our lives. For this reason, we sometimes try to avoid our fiercer emotions, believing that they will keep us from this experience of calm. But avoiding the fiery side of ourselves is denying an essential part of who we are as human beings. While we don't wish to get stuck in feelings of outrage or ferocity, these feelings serve the purpose of motivating us to right wrongs in our society, to protect those we love, and to be undeterred in pursuing our dreams. Be fiery when needed.

FALL IN LOVE WITH YOURSELF

Do you love yourself? Can you answer yes to this question without hesitation or qualifications? Without feeling egotistical or embarrassed? Many of us will consider this a very difficult question to answer. It is like being asked whether we are in love with someone we hadn't really considered loving before. It might never have occurred to us to fall in love with ourselves. But why not? We must love ourselves. If we don't, how can we expect others to love us? And how can we love others in a whole-hearted, honest way? Fall in love with yourself. It is the most meaningful love affair you can have.

CULTIVATE SLOWNESS TO CONNECT TO THE WORLD

In our society, speed is often valued over slowness. We rush through the streets whether walking or driving, text while we are talking, and send e-mails while eating. We try to get as much accomplished in as short a time as possible. We multitask endlessly because we adhere to the values of efficiency and productivity over meaningful connection. What if, for one day, we decided to value slowness? A slowness that enables us to savor the food we are eating, to connect more deeply with the people we speak with, to listen better, to look at our surroundings as we move through our day? Cultivate slowness to connect more meaningfully to the world.

JUL
2

HAVE COURAGE TO ACT ON YOUR CONVICTIONS

To have courage in the world means joining conviction to action. Being clear about your convictions, what you believe to be true and right, is the first step, but this means little unless it is joined to action. Acting on your convictions requires courage. And to be clear, having courage doesn't mean that you aren't scared; it means that despite all fear, you stand up for your beliefs even in the most challenging situation. It means that you do the right thing outwardly because you feel compelled to inwardly. What do you believe in so strongly that you will stand up and take action when needed?

BE STURDY YET RESILIENT

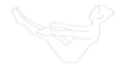

BOAT POSE
NAVASANA (NAH-VAH-sah-nah)

Sometimes the simplest-looking yoga poses are the most challenging because we must balance sturdiness and resiliency. *Navasana*, the Sanskrit name for Boat Pose, invites you to rise up into a wide V-shape that resembles a boat. Like building a boat, you must build this pose so it is strong yet yielding, flexible but solid. Resting on the back of your pelvis, lift your legs and your torso off the ground. Extend your arms in front of you, and reach your heart upward to counter the pose's downward pull. Imagine each breath is an ocean wave, and find your balance through each rise and fall.

FIND SPACIOUSNESS IN YOUR BODY

Yoga offers us the experience of spaciousness in our bodies. Spaciousness can be defined as the opposite of tightness. Tightness can take up residence in any part of our body, and when it does, we feel limited, constricted, and uncomfortable. It can be the result of tension and stress, or of muscle overuse or lack of use. Our bodies feel spacious when we loosen up the tight areas to create a greater range of motion and flexibility. We feel like we can move in ways we previously couldn't. Today, when you move on your mat, notice if you are able to create the experience of spaciousness in your body, and see how it opens up your day.

MAY THERE
BE PEACE

Om Shanti, Shanti, Shanti
(ohm SHAN-tee SHAN-tee SHAN-tee)

Peace is an internal condition before it becomes an external event. When we chant *Om Shanti, Shanti, Shanti*, a mantra that repeats the Sanskrit word for peace, we call to the peace that resides within ourselves and invite it to be pervasive in our lives. When we act peacefully, we invite more peace into our lives. We also summon peace for those around us and for the world. Just as when we act angrily at someone and receive that anger in return, when we reach out in a peaceful way, we are more likely to receive a peaceful response. The world often mirrors back to us what we offer it. Try inviting peace into your life with this mantra today.

WE SHARE A COMMON HUMANITY

When you interact with others today, remind yourself that we all share a common humanity. We move through life with human bodies, minds, and hearts. We share similar physical experiences and feel the same emotions. With each person you encounter today, try looking for the commonalities. Like you, each other person has plans, hopes, and dreams. Invite yourself to soften, accepting their dreams with the same value and reverence you hold for your own. When we recognize that we all want similar things in life, it becomes easier to be supportive of others. Our commonalities offer us lessons of compassion and support.

APPROACH THE WORLD LIKE A CHILD TO EXPERIENCE WONDER

Do you remember playing for hours with a simple object or toy when you were a child? Or finding ongoing delight in a particular picture or a specific piece of music? As young children, everything was potentially interesting. We were open to what we encountered, taking in the world with fascination and without judgment: we were deeply in touch with our sense of wonder. As we aged, we had to make decisions about our identity and our values, and while these processes were fruitful, they were often detrimental to the side of us that had such easy access to wonder. How can we stay open today? How can we hold on to our childlike curiosity about the world? Today, try to approach what you see and whomever you meet with a sense of openness and wonder. See what happens.

CONSISTENCY AND REPETITION CAN CREATE POSITIVE HABITS

To create a positive habit, we need to engage in repeated positive behavior. As we all know, it is hard to take on a new behavior and stick to it long enough for it to become natural and automatic— a habit. Begin by introducing one tiny beneficial action into your daily life. Do it at the same time every day, even marking it down in your calendar. See if you can do this action without missing a day for a month, then reevaluate. Is this behavior working for you? Does it feel natural yet? If so, move forward by introducing another small action that creates a positive shift in your daily habits. Small repeated steps taken consistently can create positive habits.

MEDITATE AT DAWN AND AT DUSK

Many believe that the most potent times to meditate are at dawn and dusk—the moments when nature is transitioning and you can most easily invite your body to follow nature's patterns. At dawn, try sitting up in bed or in a specific place for meditation in your home. In your slowly awakening state, it is easy to drop right into meditation, because your mind is halfway between your dream state and being awake and is not yet cluttered with the day's detritus. At dusk, sit in your favorite meditation place, and invite yourself to go within, just as your day slips from light into darkness. When you meditate at dawn and at dusk, you align yourself with nature, and your meditation connects you with the universe.

LOVING YOURSELF IS LOVING THE WORLD

Today, decide that your yoga practice is an offering of love to yourself. Many of us find that loving ourselves is a difficult thing to do, as if it were somehow self-indulgent or wrong to feel love for our own selves. But the reality is that in order to be able to love others, we need to begin by loving ourselves. How can we offer love to other people when we can't feel it within ourselves? Today, invite your yoga practice to become an affirmation of self-love, a way of treating yourself with the same love and attention that you might offer to another. Loving yourself is loving the world.

TWIST GENTLY TO CREATE POWERFUL CHANGE

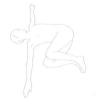

RECLINING ABDOMINAL TWIST POSE
JATHARA PARIVARTANASANA (jah-tah-rah pah-
ree-var-tah-NAH-sah-nah)

Twisting yoga poses invite movement and openness into parts of the body that are otherwise difficult to access. Lie on your back. Bend your knees to your chest, and twist from the waist, releasing your knees to one side and opening up the top side of the body from the shoulder to the outer pelvis. This enables you to shift your muscles, organs, and skin in a way that is sometimes elusive in other poses. It is often the subtle movements, choices, and decisions in our lives that create powerful change. This gentle but powerful opening, which is often done toward the end of a yoga practice session, relaxes us deeply and readies us for our final poses.

JUL
12

COMPASSION FOR OTHERS IS COMPASSION FOR YOURSELF

How critical are you toward others? How hard are you on yourself? We often criticize in others what we like least in ourselves. Notice what you find yourself critiquing in other people. Ask yourself: *When do I notice this quality or habit in myself?* Then instead of resisting, try to soften and look more compassionately at your own imperfections and at the imperfections of others. If you find that you can't change the habit or tendency, choose to accept it and manage it in a way that does not negatively affect your life. Having compassion for the imperfections of others is also having compassion for yourself.

BEGIN THE REST OF YOUR LIFE AT THIS MOMENT

Everything that has brought you to this very moment has made you who you are—the good and bad, the triumphs and tragedies. Here you are in this place, at this moment in time, which is the point of departure for the rest of your life. Today, ask yourself: *How do I wish to begin the rest of my life right now? Which choices will I make again? Which aspects of my life do I want to change? Who do I need to thank? What do I need to walk away from?* With honor for your past, move forward into the future. You begin the rest of your life at this moment.

THE MYTH OF PARVATI AND GANESHA

The goddess Parvati was lonely because her husband, the god Shiva, was away meditating in the mountains. She waited days, weeks, and eventually years for him to return, but still, he meditated. Parvati wished that she could conceive a child so that the child could keep her company, but of course, she couldn't conceive since her beloved was absent. One day, as she was thinking this over, she had a realization: since Shiva lived within her heart, he was actually always present. Laughing with delight, she began to rub her arms, legs, and belly, and from her laughter and the oils of her skin, she created her son Ganesha. This myth reminds us that by turning within, we can recognize our innate power and capabilities.

YOGA ENABLES US TO ACCESS SPIRIT

Yoga opens up the creaky corners of our bodies. Our muscles soften and lengthen, and we feel more powerful through the openness that we begin to experience. When we feel open, we can more readily tap into something that we often call spirit—a feeling or sensation that shapes our dreams and our connection with the greater world. To access our spiritual selves, we need to tend to our physical selves, because body and spirit are not separate. Yoga keeps our bodies open, enabling us to access spirit.

LEARNING TO LISTEN
TO OURSELVES

JUL
15

Just like we learn from listening to other people's thoughts and ideas, we also learn from listening to ourselves. Listening to ourselves is different from listening to others: to listen to ourselves, we have to become settled enough to let our thoughts rise to the surface of our consciousness. Just as we have to be quiet in a conversation to hear what the other person has to say, we have to quiet ourselves to hear our own deeper layers of thought. Inside our minds, there is ongoing chatter and buzz. When we quiet our minds, we can tap into our dreams, desires, and intuition. Find some time today to slow down and listen to the parts of you that speak the most quietly.

YOGA IS: AN EXPRESSION OF BEAUTY

Yoga poses have a functional purpose, in that they offer us strength, openness, and invigoration, but yoga poses are also artful. Each individual pose has a name and is a specific physical expression of beauty. The poses do not have to be extreme or acrobatic to convey this beauty: it is the attitude the yoga practitioner brings to the poses that shapes the quality of their expression. Ask yourself: *Today, how can I make my yoga practice into an expression of beauty?* Even if you only do one pose, do it with focus and dedication. Try dedicating it to someone or something you love, and from the inside out, create beauty.

GROUND YOURSELF TO GO WITHIN

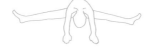

WIDE-ANGLE SEATED FORWARD BEND POSE
UPAVISTHA KONASANA (oo-pah-vish-tah koh-
NAH-sah-nah)

It is only when you are very grounded that you can slow down and go within. *Upavistha Konasana,* the Sanskrit name for Wide-Angle Seated Forward Bend Pose, offers this deep experience of stability. The backs of your legs and the base of your pelvis are settled into the ground, supporting you. This solidity enables you to move and shift in the upper body, as you open your legs wide, bend at the waist, and extend forward to prop yourself up on your hands or forearms. Close your eyes. Breathe. As you fold forward toward the ground, allow yourself to find an inner sense of quiet.

FIND THE HUMOR IN LIFE

Try to laugh every day. Humor gives us perspective on the world and on ourselves. The more we cultivate a sense of humor, the better equipped we are to tackle stressful situations and maintain a relaxed state of mind. Many studies have demonstrated how amusement and laughter are beneficial to our health and well-being. Laughter can disperse tension. Humor can shift our heavier emotional states. Each day, seek out humor through your friends and acquaintances, through reading, and in the media. And most important, bring a sense of humor to the events of your daily life.

EXPRESS YOUR GRATITUDE AND TRANSFORM YOUR EXPERIENCE OF THE WORLD

If you want to transform your experience of the world, express your gratitude. Try this as a practice today: Offer thanks to all the people who offer you kindness or a service. If a door is held for you, say thank you. If you buy coffee, express your thanks to the person who made it and sold it to you. In gratitude for any small gesture, use your words to bring the energy of gratitude into the world in an active way. Write a message of appreciation to someone, letting them know how much you value them. Say it. Write it. Express it in every way you can. Check in with yourself before you go to sleep, asking yourself, *How did it feel to be a generator of gratitude in the world today?*

WALKING
MEDITATION

Incorporate a walking meditation into your day today. You can either choose to go for a walk or you can do it on your way to work or when you are running errands. Focus on each step you take, mindfully placing one foot down in front of the other and noticing the way your foot connects to the ground. There are three main points of contact in the sole of the foot, so see if with every step, you can roll from the heel to the little toe mound to the big toe mound, making equal contact with each of the three points. Let your movement be smooth and even, and invite that equilibrium to resonate in the rest of your body. Notice whether allowing yourself to focus on the basic workings of your feet and body can offer you tranquility and wonder.

YOU ARE AN EXQUISITELY MADE STRUCTURE

Draw your attention to the bones of your body. Begin by moving your awareness from skin through muscle, tissues, and fluid to arrive at your skeletal system. The bones connect and attach in all sorts of ways. Like the architecture of a building, your frame stacks and balances, bends and pivots. It is an amazing design formed by a beautiful and graceful network of shapes and attachments. Right now make a basic movement, such as lifting an arm or a leg, taking a step, or shifting in your seat. Notice all the ways in which the framework of your body is capable of moving. Notice how one central repositioning of your hips or spine creates an entire series of auxiliary movements throughout the architecture of your body. You are an exquisitely made structure.

THE MYTH OF DURGA, THE BUFFALO-DEMON SLAYER

The demon Mahisha, who had once received a blessing of invulnerability to men and gods, was on a rampage, conquering and killing. Fearful of Mahisha's invulnerability, the gods turned to the great goddess Parvati for help. Parvati agreed to battle Mahisha, so the gods equipped her with all of their powers and weapons. This transformed her into the great warrior goddess Durga. The battle began. Mahisha changed himself into a lion, a man, and an elephant, in order to attack in different ways. Finally, he took the form of a buffalo and lunged at Durga's pet lion. Enraged, she lopped off the buffalo's neck, and out crawled Mahisha in his demon form. She picked up the trident of her beloved, the god Shiva, and plunged it into Mahisha, vanquishing him and freeing the world from his tyranny. Like Durga, what do you need to vanquish in order for you and your world to thrive? How will you tap into your inner power—and the power around you—to do so?

LET YOUR BREATH BE YOUR TEACHER

If you want to learn about yourself, observe your breath. Check in. Is your breath short or long? Hurried or calm? Simply observing your breath can indicate how you are feeling at any particular moment. If the breath is short and abrupt, it may signify that you need to lengthen or deepen it in order to relax or feel invigorated. If deep breathing is agitating you, you may need to let the breath become shallow in order to calm yourself. Get quiet. Listen to what your breath is telling you. Let your breath be your teacher.

DEVELOP DAILY RITUALS
TO ENRICH YOUR LIFE

Our days are enriched when we participate in
rituals that help create meaning, making our lives
fuller and more rewarding. These rituals can be
as simple as lighting a candle, saying a morning
prayer, or setting an intention at the beginning
of the day. We can bless our food before we eat
or take a moment to write a daily gratitude list.
When we engage in simple daily rituals, we direct
our attention more fully to what is meaningful.
Through this process, our lives feel fuller and
more satisfying. Today, create and participate
in a personal ritual that celebrates something
you value in your life.

YOGA IS: A GIFT TO YOURSELF

Your yoga practice can be a celebration of your daily life as well as a means of support through challenging times. By choosing to practice yoga, you are choosing to care for yourself by strengthening your body, supporting your heart, and easing your mind. Think of the delight of giving a gift to someone you love. Offer your practice to yourself in this same loving spirit. Accept the benefits your practice offers you with receptivity and grace. When you step onto your mat today, enjoy your role as the giver of the gift and as its recipient.

MAINTAINING HEALTHY PERSONAL BOUNDARIES

Yoga enables us to become more accepting of different people and situations in our lives. There are times when welcoming a new situation into our lives is positive, but other times when it may be inappropriate or may threaten our well-being. Honoring our personal space and valuing our individual integrity is as important as being open. Yoga develops our awareness, and we need to use that awareness to discern what is healthy and unhealthy for us. There are times to say yes, to open our lives to new people and unexpected situations, but there are also times to say no, to use our wisdom and insight to create and maintain healthy personal boundaries in our lives.

CONNECT TO YOUR WISDOM

Jnana Mudra (NYAH-nah MOO-drah)
Mudra of Wisdom

Each moment of your day is an opportunity to learn about yourself and about your world. *Jnana* is the Sanskrit word for knowledge. Today, form *Jnana Mudra*, a hand gesture signifying your engagement with your learning process. When you rest the backs of your hands on your thighs, and lift your index fingers to touch your thumbs, you form *Jnana Mudra*, the gesture of knowledge. *Jnana Mudra* connects you more deeply to your knowledge and to your process of acquiring it. It demonstrates that you value the life experiences that offer you wisdom.

ALIGN WITH NATURE TO ALIGN WITH YOURSELF

When we turn our attention toward nature, we become more closely aligned with it. We remember that we, too, are nature, and then we begin to see that there are parallels between what we see around us and our own experiences. We notice the ways in which our energy patterns rise and fall with the weather and with the seasons. We notice growth and transformation, such as a plant sprouting, blossoming, and withering, and we realize that this is always happening in our lives as well. Recognizing our connectivity to nature is a step toward becoming more attuned to our environment and to ourselves. When we align with nature, we become more attuned to everything that is living, and we begin to live more aware and harmonious lives.

THE TRUTH WILL
SET YOU FREE

When you tell the truth, you have nothing to hide.
This is liberating. Even when the truth is embar-
rassing or painful, denying it doesn't get rid of the
discomfort; it only suppresses it, so that it lurks
in the back closet of your mind and heart. One
untruth usually initiates a series of untruths since
you need to tell more and more lies to cover up
the initial lie. When the truth is out in the open, that
space behind you is free. There is nothing unsaid
lurking behind you. You are free from the tyranny
of untruths, half-truths, and denial. Telling the truth
will set you free.

RELEASE
TO RELAX

By releasing tension, we find relaxation. Think about the ways in which tension manifests in our bodies: a tight jaw, a clenched back, a sore neck. Yoga can help release the physical discomfort resulting from stress and tension. It is a powerful way to address the effects of sadness, anger, and anxiety on the body. The more we move, the better we shift the stuck energy, stiffness, and tension that may have caused it. Join breath to movement: do yoga to release and relax.

DO THE INNER WORK SO
YOU CAN FLOURISH

To grow as a person, you have to do the inner work—
that is, learning about yourself and deciding who
you want to be in the world so you can change what
needs to be changed and evolve as a person. Good
starting points are yoga, meditation, or anything
that draws you into a state of focused contemplation about your life. Inner work involves asking
yourself tough questions about what you value
and how you wish to be in the world. You have to
dive down into the muck of what you don't want
to look at in yourself in order to excavate your
insecurities and fears. Only then can you deal with
them. This acknowledgment begins your process
of release and of personal growth.

FIND
MOTIVATION

We all need motivation to achieve things in our lives, but how can we become motivated? Start by thinking about what inspires you: the people you love, the causes you find meaningful, the things that make your day more beautiful and more uplifting. Then choose one of them to be your day's motivator. Over the course of your day, keep returning to that motivator, and imagine your actions serving it. By honoring something outside ourselves, we have a sense of purpose. We are motivated to follow through with our vision.

BEING STRAIGHTFORWARD IN OUR BODIES AND IN OUR LIVES

STAFF POSE
DANDASANA (dahn-DAH-sah-nah)

It can be difficult to be straightforward with the people around us. Being straightforward requires a firm commitment to ourselves and our beliefs, and a commitment to honesty in our interactions with others. Yoga can help us maintain these commitments. *Dandasana*, the Sanskrit term for Staff Pose, invites us to be firm and resolute in our posture, so that we experience clarity and directness in our bodies. Seated on the ground with your legs stretched out in front of you, lift from your tailbone to the top of your head. Rest your fingertips on the ground by your hips. As you practice this pose, consider how the straightforward positioning of your body can translate to your thoughts, words, and interactions.

FINDING THE SACRED IN NATURE

If you treat nature with reverence, the natural world becomes sacred. As you move through your day today, try noticing and connecting with the natural objects around you, whether you are in nature or in a city. Examine a plant more closely than you have before, noticing the intricacy of its form and leaves. Pick up a stone or a piece of fruit, and feel its particular shape and texture. Every part of nature is deserving of our wonderment and reverence. If you seek out the sacred in nature, you will find it. And as a part of nature, we too are sacred.

CELEBRATE YOURSELF

Today, celebrate yourself. No matter what is going on, how busy you are, and whatever challenges you may be facing, let today be a celebration of you. Begin by listing ten things that you love about yourself: recent successes, personal accomplishments, your favorite aspects of your personality, and the admirable qualities that you possess. Write them down, and then congratulate yourself on each of them. Throughout your day, refer to this list. Inwardly compliment yourself as if you were receiving a compliment from a friend, family member, or coworker. Bask in the light of your own personal celebration of you.

ACCESS THE PRIMAL POWER OF YOUR FEROCITY

Om Kali Ma
(ohm KAH-lee mah)

We contain both gentleness and ferocity. We often associate ferocity with something negative, since it is frightening, uncontrolled, and primal. But while ferocity may sometimes be an unattractive quality, it is essential to surviving in the world and to protecting those we love. *Om Kali Ma* is a mantra we can chant to invoke our ferocity. *Om* evokes everything that exists, *Kali* is the most ferocious of goddesses, and *Ma* means divine mother. When we are pushed to our limit, when someone we love is imperiled, or when we need to defend ourselves, we can chant *Om Kali Ma* to access the primal power of ferocity within us.

WANDER AND YOU
WILL FIND BEAUTY

Right now, think about the experience of wandering through a new landscape or exploring an enormous building you've never entered that offers you surprises at every turn. Tap into the sensation of opening to the unexpected, of having no idea what you will see and discover. When you let your body or mind roam, you open to life. When you wander, you discover new perspectives and ideas. Your thoughts become less constrained and more open to creativity. Today, let your body wander. Or if you cannot do that, let your mind wander. By releasing a little control, you allow life to present itself to you in diverse and beautiful new ways.

UNPLUG AND EXPERIENCE THE WORLD MORE FULLY

Plan ahead for a day in which you can unplug
entirely—meaning no phone, no computer, no
television. For one entire day, commit to being
electronics-free. This may involve getting away
from your home and your usual habits, or you may
choose to keep your daily routine but without your
phone, computer, and television. Make a plan for
what you will do that day. You may wish to spend
time with friends, go for a long walk, read, cook,
or do something creative. When we put aside our
attachment to electronics and the media, we open
our senses more fully to the world. So even for one
day, unplug, and see what happens.

ALIGN YOURSELF: BODY, MIND, AND HEART

There are three major components to creating alignment in your life: your body, your mind, and your heart. The three are interdependent, so by caring for one, you indirectly care for the others, which contributes to your sense of alignment. Envision a triangle. When one angle is pulled out of alignment, the entire triangle becomes misaligned. In the same way, when you neglect your body, your mind, or your heart, you become misaligned. Yoga can help you create and maintain alignment. It opens your body, which creates ease in your heart and mind. It relaxes your thinking, which releases tension and anxiety in your body and heart. It opens your heart, which helps you find comfort in your body and mind. Align yourself: body, mind, and heart.

CULTIVATE INNER PEACE

Finding inner peace can require work. This work takes two forms: effort and release. It takes effort because if we want to experience a peaceful state of mind, we must first decide that we want it. Then we must arrange our lives around obtaining it. This may mean taking steps such as creating a regular yoga or meditation practice and choosing to spend our time with people who support this way of thinking. Cultivating inner peace also takes release because we need to do the work of letting go of whatever is blocking us from experiencing peace. We have to relinquish thoughts that don't serve us, from old ideas and conceptions of who we are to what we think we want. We have to give up habits and beliefs that we have been holding on to for years. Through effort and release, we are freed from what has held us back, and we find the peace of self-acceptance.

MEDITATE ON
TOUCH

Today, try meditating on the bodily sensation of touch. You can do this at any time and in any place. Either close your eyes or simply soften your gaze. Begin observing your breath, feeling the air as it enters in through your nostrils or mouth, and then the sensation of your breath releasing. Direct your attention to the air touching your skin wherever it is exposed, noticing whether it is warm or cold, still or moving. Feel the texture of your clothing against your skin, and the firmness or softness of the ground beneath you. Let yourself float in this state of heightened awareness, appreciating your body's experience of touch.

WHAT DO YOU REVERE?

What do you revere? What consistently inspires devotion in you? What lifts your heart? What generates feelings of awe or gratitude and makes you feel like giving thanks every time you encounter it? A place? A piece of music? Something in nature? An artwork? These are the things you should return to when you need the life-affirming feelings of awe or reverence. All of us should have the chance to regularly experience these feelings, since they make life meaningful, inspirational, and moving. Reverence inspires us.

YOUR BODY IS LIKE A WAVE

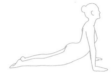

UPWARD-FACING DOG POSE
URDHVA MUKHA SVANASANA
(oor-dvah moo-kah shvah-NAH-sah-nah)

When you practice *Urdhva Mukha Svanasana*, the Sanskrit name for Upward-Facing Dog Pose, your body curls up and forward like a wave, evoking the suspended moment just before a wave crashes. To arrange your body in this yoga pose, lie on your belly with your palms planted on the ground by your chest. Lift your torso, draw your shoulders back, and reach your heart toward the sky. Your body weight is balanced between your palms and the tops of your feet, and your collarbones are wide open. In a moment, the wave will subside as you release back down and proceed to the next pose. But for now, in Upward-Facing Dog, simply open and pause.

FORGIVENESS BENEFITS YOU

How can you forgive when you feel wronged? It is helpful to begin by recognizing that holding on to anger and resentment may damage you more than it does anyone else. Think of the ways in which these feelings often manifest in the body: a clenched jaw, tight muscles, an upset stomach, and the overall wear and tear of tension and stress. Forgiveness is tough, especially if you feel wronged or slighted. But the process of recognizing when anger and resentment rise up inside of you, noticing how detrimental the effects of these emotions are within you, and then consciously releasing these emotions again and again is key to your individual well-being. Choosing to forgive releases damaging feelings and affirms your dedication to your own self-care. In this way, the act of forgiveness is an embrace of yourself, an assertion that your current state of well-being is more of a priority than a challenging past event. Forgiveness benefits you and forgiveness heals.

HELP PEOPLE TO
FEEL SEEN

Today, look at people. Listen to people. Acknowledge someone you don't generally acknowledge:
thank someone, smile at someone. Thank the
person who holds a door for you, the driver of the
bus, someone who serves you food, the person you
pass by every day on your way to work but you have
never said hello to. Help make people feel visible.
Recognize, connect, and appreciate. Let people
know that they count by making them feel seen and
heard. Try this affirming practice today, and feel
how rewarding it is to be appreciative of the people
you encounter in your daily life.

THE MYTH OF HANUMAN'S HEART

The battle between the great god Ram and the demon Ravana, who had kidnapped Ram's beloved goddess Sita, was over. Sita, Ram, and the people of their kingdom were celebrating. In gratitude to Hanuman, the monkey god who was the hero of the battle and their cherished friend, Sita unclasped the jewels from her neck and gave them to him. But instead of thanking her, Hanuman scrutinized the necklace and began pulling it apart. As everyone watched in shock, he held each gem up to the light. He explained, "I am looking for the presence of Sita and Ram in each gem, because they are what is truly of value." Some people laughed, skeptical of the extent of Hanuman's devotion. In response, Hanuman dug his fingers into the center of his rib cage and opened it up to reveal his heart. Inscribed on his heart was a picture of Sita and Ram, pulsing with devotion. Hanuman's devotion reminds us to ask ourselves: *What do we value so deeply that it is inscribed on our heart?*

RECOGNIZE YOUR CONNECTION TO THE UNIVERSE TO EXPERIENCE ONENESS

Our bodies meet the rest of the universe where our skin ends. All that delineates our bodies from their surroundings is this thin layer. Try releasing the idea that we are separate or apart from everything else that exists, and instead, try looking for the connections. We can assert our unique individuality while still recognizing that we are deeply interconnected. We are one elaborate tapestry made up of infinite interwoven threads. We are many and we are one. When we recognize our connection with the universe, we have the ecstatic experience of oneness.

YOGA IS: SERVING YOUR HEART

Our bodies and our hearts are intricately connected. When we release tension and pain in the
body, we often release it in the heart as well. By
nurturing both the body and the heart, we can
more easily experience contentment and joy. Yoga
opens up our bodies, which opens up our hearts.
If our hearts are ill at ease—for example, if we are
feeling upset, challenged, or closed off—we can
practice yoga to create a shift. The next time your
heart feels ill at ease, try moving on your mat and
see what happens.

AWARENESS GIVES ACCESS TO BEAUTY

If we are open to experiencing beauty, it will present itself. Beauty comes in an infinite number of forms, and our conception of it can be continually upended by encountering it in new ways. To experience beauty in all of its diversity, we need to cultivate our awareness, which involves more listening, more watching, and a greater overall attentiveness in our daily lives. Imagine if you had just one idea of what a beautiful flower was and someone presented you with a different flower. Would you find it ugly or would you allow yourself to welcome it in a new awareness of what beauty can be? Awareness offers us ways to expand our limited conception of things. It challenges our fixed definitions and offers us access to infinite beauty.

ENGAGE YOUR ENTIRE BODY ON YOUR MAT

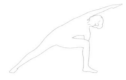

SIDE ANGLE POSE
PARSVAKONASANA (par-shva-koh-NAH-sah-nah)

How fully engaged can you be in any given moment? In *Parsvakonasana*, the Sanskrit name for Side Angle Pose, each of your four limbs is exploring a different shape and direction. Your front knee is bent, your back leg is extended, one arm reaches toward the ground, and the other arm extends up over your head. Your body is fully engaged in a range of simultaneous movements and gestures when you form *Parsvakonasana*. The effect of the pose on your body is a diverse series of satisfying stretches and openings, dynamically engaging your full attention as you arrange yourself in the pose, hold it, and then release it.

SIT WITH ANGER

The next time you feel anger, pause for a moment. Shift your focus from the object of your anger, and begin to explore what anger feels like in your body. In what parts of your body does the anger seem to be located? Your jaw? Your chest? Your hands? And what, specifically, does the sensation of anger feel like? Take a mental step back and look at the anger: Does it have a color? A particular texture? A quality of sound? How does this intense emotion resonate physically within your body? Sometimes by experiencing as much as we can of a negative emotion, we can begin to understand it, and shift our experience so that it loosens its grip on us.

GIVE THANKS
WHEN YOU EAT

Before you begin to eat your meals today, pause to give thanks. Imagine all of the work involved in getting that food onto your plate. Think of nature: the seasons and the soil. Imagine the people who have worked to plant, cultivate, and grow your food. Also consider the people who have harvested, packed, and delivered this food to the place where you bought it. Think about who served you or helped you in purchasing your food. All of this recognition only takes a few seconds, but the difference it makes in the way you eat and experience your food is tremendous. You have chosen to bring your consciousness to one of your essential everyday acts. You have chosen to feel gratitude in your daily life.

MEDITATION IS EASIER THAN YOU THINK

Meditation is easier that you think. We read so much about how to practice meditation, about meditation classes and retreats, and about the importance of beginning a meditation practice. Still, though, many of us don't know where or how to begin. We somehow think that meditation is a carefully honed skill or that there is some trick to doing it. This makes beginning a meditation practice feel elusive or daunting. We can begin by simply sitting and watching our thoughts arise, focusing on our breath, or silently repeating a word. Embracing slowness and focusing in these ways can give us access to a meditative state right now.

TREAT YOUR FEET
WITH LOVE

Consider the soles of your feet as miniature maps of the body, different areas representing connections to different organs and body parts. Remember this when you choose a pair of shoes, when you spend a long time standing, and when you wash and care for your feet. Offer the soles of your feet some extra attention, massaging, pumicing, and oiling them. Your feet support your entire body weight when standing, and form your connection to the earth when you run and walk. So, imagine the extra care they need to be happy and healthy. Treat your feet with love.

A MYTH OF KRISHNA AND THE MILKMAIDS IN THE FOREST

One day, the beautiful god Krishna began to play his flute at the edge of the forest. All of the milkmaids in the cow-herding town where he lived were madly in love with Krishna, and were seduced by the sound of his music. They abandoned their milking and butter churning and wandered deep into the forest in search of him. Arriving at a lake, the milkmaids shed their brightly colored saris to bathe in the cooling waters. In their love-struck state, they didn't notice Krishna gathering up their clothing and climbing up into the tree, where he began to call their names and tease them. The milkmaids just gazed up at him and smiled, intoxicated with love. This myth invites you to see your heart as the forest. Wander into it and lose yourself in love.

BREATHE INTO YOUR BONES

Our bones are deeply connected to our breath. What does this mean? The marrow of our bones thrives on oxygen. So with each breath, our bones are supported and sustained. Take a deep breath right now and imagine that you are breathing directly into your bones: your shoulder blades, collarbones, rib cage, pelvis, spine, and skull, and the bones of your arms and hands, legs and feet. Imagine filling your entire skeletal system with energy that radiates outward, from your bones through your body. With each breath you take, you nourish yourself.

LET YOUR DAILY YOGA PRACTICE BE A REFUGE

Many of us begin practicing yoga as a way to relieve stress and find a sense of inner peace. When times get tough, we know that going to a yoga class or practicing even a few poses on our own can tip the balance toward ease once again or at least alleviate the intensity of whatever we are going through. This week, see if you can treat your yoga practice as a refuge, a place of ease and release that is always available to you. All you need to do is step through its door. Even the slightest effort toward practice will offer you access to this place, and knowing that it is there will support your heart.

ARE YOUR THOUGHTS ELEVATING YOU OR DRAGGING YOU DOWN?

Our ways of thinking feel like second nature, but if we look closely, we can begin to notice some thought patterns that help us and others that hurt us. Today, observe your habitual thought patterns. Notice if your inner conversation is elevating and encouraging or is negative and defeatist. Each time you find yourself in a negative place, ask yourself: *Is this really how I want to make myself feel? How could I change my attitude about this situation so it would be more affirming for me?* Then speak to yourself as if you were talking to a valued friend. Encourage yourself to choose to move away from patterns that are negative and to emphasize your ways of thinking that are positive and uplifting for you.

THE MYTH OF HANUMAN MISTAKING THE SUN FOR A MANGO

When the beloved monkey god Hanuman was a baby, he looked up into the sky and saw the sun god Surya whom he mistook for a giant glowing mango. He leapt through the air to try to eat him. The powerful god Indra witnessed this and, panicking, he threw a thunderbolt at Hanuman to stop him. The thunderbolt struck the little monkey in the jaw and sent him crashing to the ground. Hanuman's father, the wind god Vayu, was irate. Cradling Hanuman in his arms, he angrily began to suck all the air out of the world. To appease Vayu, Indra and the other gods apologized, healed Hanuman's jaw, and revived him. At Vayu's insistence, they all gave Hanuman magical powers. From that point on, Hanuman was invulnerable in battle, incapable of being hurt by either fire or water, and had the ability to shape-shift. This myth shows us that, like Hanuman, it is often through our accidents and mistakes that we grow, gaining wisdom and power.

FOCUS ON ONE TASK AT A TIME TO ACHIEVE BALANCE

Balance can feel elusive in daily life. Work and to-do lists can consume our days, making us feel like there is no time for family, self-care, or relaxation. The best way to approach a seemingly insurmountable workload is to create a plan, focus on one task at a time, and work at it until it is finished. Then move on to the next task. In this way, you quiet your mind by focusing it, keeping it from leaping ahead to all the other things you need to do. If you can fix your attention on what you are doing at any given moment, you can live more fully in the present, deriving more satisfaction from what you are actually accomplishing, and feeling more balanced throughout your day.

APPRECIATE WHAT YOU HAVE TO EXPERIENCE CONTENTMENT

The experience of contentment can emerge from a mindset of appreciation for what we have, who we are, and where we are in the world. We spend much of our time focused on accomplishing new things, looking for new opportunities, and moving toward our future—all of which are important to our growth. But it is equally important to pause and take a moment to simply appreciate what we have. This doesn't mean that we stop growing. We can experience contentment while continuing to evolve as individuals. In fact, our growth is often more satisfying when we regularly experience contentment by appreciating what we have.

FIND
QUIETUDE

Regardless of what may be happening in the outside world, we can find a certain calm and stillness
within. Quietude is a quality that we can nurture
and grow through our yoga and meditation practices. The movement of our bodies during our yoga
practice helps us relax. The practice of meditation
helps us focus our minds. When these two practices
are a part of our daily lives, they help maintain our
inner equilibrium, so that we have a place to go when
the outer world is loud and disruptive. Our yoga
and meditation practices are the gardeners of our
quietude.

MEDITATE ON YOUR GOALS AND DESIRES

Today, during a quiet moment, close your eyes and envision what you want to do in your life—your hopes and dreams. Imagine yourself in a state of having already achieved it all. Notice what achieving your dreams feels like in your body. Notice what it feels like for your heart and mind. Sometimes, envisioning these feelings of accomplishment can help pave the way to success, because it mentally and emotionally prepares us for manifesting our dreams. Envisioning sets the stage and helps us feel that our goals are within our reach. Sometimes we need to close our eyes to see farther. Each morning this week, try an envisioning exercise and see how it sets the tone for your day.

BE READY FOR TRANSITIONS

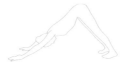

DOWNWARD-FACING DOG POSE

ADHO MUKHA SVANASANA (ah-dho moo-kah shvah-NAH-sah-nah)

With your palms planted on your mat, your hips stretched up and back, and your legs rooted to the ground through your feet, you form *Adho Mukha Svanasana*, the Sanskrit name for Downward-Facing Dog. This yoga pose is one from which you can easily move into almost any other pose; for example, you can step forward into a Forward Bend, glide forward into Plank Pose, or fold back gently into Child's Pose. It is a pose of transition—a pose in which you can pause and gather yourself before moving or shifting your weight in another direction. Practice Downward-Facing Dog and meet transitions with grace.

MAKE YOUR HOME A SANCTUARY

Whether you live in a sizable house or a tiny apartment, make it your own. Your home can be the outward manifestation of your personality, reflecting your likes and preferences. Create a home for yourself that takes the form of an external expression of your innermost self. When you walk into your home, you will feel happy, peaceful, and energized. Any place can be made to feel welcoming with a little care and attention to detail. When your home reflects your best self, you will have created a sanctuary for yourself. Your care for your surroundings offers you refuge. Make your home your sanctuary.

BELIEVE IN YOURSELF TO OVERCOME SELF-DOUBT

Doubt can stem from our wisdom or can result from our having a clear perspective on things. When we have doubts, we aren't just believing what we have been told; we are applying our intellect and our critical thinking to our life experiences. But excessive self-doubt can be crippling. It can undermine our desire and ability to make choices and take action. It is essential to believe in ourselves. By affirming our thoughts and ideas, we prevent self-doubt from immobilizing us. We thrive when we find a balance between listening to our misgivings and knowing when to push them aside, assert ourselves, and take action.

I AM
THAT

So'ham
(soh-hahm)

The mantra *So'ham* is the natural sound of the
breath—your inhale making the sound of *So* and
your exhale making the sound of *Ham*. *So'ham*
means I am that, signifying the recognition when
we see reflections of ourselves in the world and the
world within ourselves. We are a product not just
of our DNA, but of every experience we have ever
had, our environment, and every person we have
known. When you move through the world today,
recognize that everyone and everything around
you shows you something about yourself. Say this
mantra to yourself. *So'ham*. I am that. As you do
so, see how your relationship with the world around
you shifts and deepens.

COMMUNITY
MATTERS

We are social beings. We are more engaged with the world when we can regularly share the company of others. And we especially benefit from being around people who both elevate us and keep us real. The Sanskrit word for a community that we choose to join is *kula* (KOO-lah). The term is often applied to a yoga community, but we can use it to refer to any community formed through shared experience or particular interests. In a *kula*, we surround ourselves with people who respect our ideas and support our dreams, people who affirm us but also can offer suggestions and constructive criticism. To be a member of a community means to give and to receive respectful truth and encouragement.

CHALLENGING CONVERSATIONS CAN TRANSFORM RELATIONSHIPS

Take a moment to reflect on your relationships. Is there a difficult but necessary conversation you are delaying or avoiding? Is there something you want to express to someone but are holding back because of the potential discomfort you may feel, or fear of what it might bring about? When we avoid a challenging conversation in any relationship, we make things worse. Silencing our thoughts and suppressing what needs to be said can cause the issue to eat away at us and make us angry or resentful. It can be the toughest thing to do, but when we know it's the right thing to do, we must choose to communicate. The conversation might be messy and upsetting, and the issue may or may not be easily resolved, but communication can shift what you are feeling, change your perspective, and transform your relationship.

BREATHE TO BE STEADY WHEN YOUR WORLD IS CHANGING

In times of great change when you don't feel in control, how do you regain your steadiness so you feel balanced? To keep from panicking, try to tap into the stillness at your center. You can do this by focusing on your breath. Begin by closing or softening your gaze and drawing your attention inward, away from whatever distractions may be in your surroundings. You may also encounter distractions in your thoughts. Draw your attention away from them and focus on the steady rise and fall of your breath inside your body. The consistent rhythm of this rise and fall is reassuring, and can offer you access to a deep sense of stillness at your center. Remind yourself that regardless of what may be happening in your life, you can find steadiness and calm through the consistent movement of your breath.

MEDITATE TO UNCLUTTER YOUR MIND

When we feel bombarded by our thoughts, we can unclutter our minds by practicing a simple meditation. The next time you feel bombarded, sit and close your eyes. Notice the thoughts that enter your mind. Instead of engaging with each thought—analyzing it, creating associations, and letting feelings arise around it—remain detached from the thought and observe it as it floats by. Do this with each thought that enters your mind, giving it a little nod of acknowledgment and allowing it to drift along. Today, try this several times, and notice how the process offers you a calmer, less cluttered mind.

DEVOTION CAN SHAPE YOUR LIFE

Devotion is both a feeling and an act. When we are devoted to someone or something, we move through the world with that person or thing in our heart. The feeling of devotion is deep reverence and love. We feel inspired and emotionally full. The feeling of devotion directs our actions and behavior, helping us decide what is important and make decisions based on those values. Devotion connects us to something greater than ourselves. Today, think about who or what inspires your devotion. Ask yourself: *How does that devotion help shape my life?*

BE FOCUSED AND
UNDETERRED IN LIFE

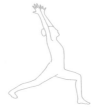

WARRIOR I POSE
VIRABHADRASANA I (VI-rah-bah-DRA-sah-nah)

How do you prepare yourself for engaging with life's challenges? To face challenges, we must be focused and undeterred. Access these qualities within yourself through *Virabhadrasana I*, the Sanskrit name for Warrior I pose. Take a wide and powerful stance, turning your back heel down with the foot angled forward. Face out resolutely over your bent front leg, while extending your arms toward the sky on either side of your head. The word *vira* means hero or warrior, or to be fully and wholeheartedly engaged with life. *Vira I* is a complex pose in which your body must root down while twisting forward and reaching upward.

UNCOVER YOUR CREATIVE SELF

Within each of us there is a creative self. This creative self can take many different forms because creativity is a quality that can be cultivated, not an inborn trait that only certain people possess. To uncover your creativity, ask yourself: *Where do I desire creativity in my life? Do I want to be innovative in my job or at home? Do I wish to uncover my creative self through writing, music, art, or my yoga practice?* First, become aware of what you are already doing creatively in various areas. Then, brainstorm as many different and unexpected choices for creativity that you can come up with for yourself. Open yourself to experimentation and, through trial and error, let your creative self emerge and develop.

SET AN INTENTION FOR YOUR YOGA PRACTICE

Setting an intention for your yoga practice can be as simple as dedicating your practice to someone or to something greater than yourself. Through the process, you honor that person or cause. Your intention creates a point of reference to which you return repeatedly as you move, keeping you centered, focused, and aligned with the subject of your intention. Much as we make a toast to celebrate someone, or make a donation in someone else's name, setting an intention is an act of honoring, whether it be a person who has impacted your life positively or a cause such as world peace. The act of setting an intention connects you to the greater world. It makes your yoga practice bigger and more meaningful. It honors both the subject of your intention and you for having offered it.

THE MYTH OF GANESHA LOSING HIS HEAD TO GAIN HIS GREATNESS

One morning, the goddess Parvati asked her son Ganesha to guard the door to their home so she could rest. Soon, a man emerged from the forest. He had long, matted dreadlocks, wore nothing but a tiger skin, and was covered with sacred ash. It was the powerful god Shiva, Ganesha's father, who was finally returning home after years of meditating in the mountains. He demanded entry, but Ganesha, who was born after his father had left, refused. They did not recognize each other. Enraged, Shiva lopped off his own son's head. Parvati rushed out, horrified, and sent Shiva into the forest with Ganesha's uncles to find their son a new head. The first creature they encountered was an elephant, who, recognizing the gods' greatness, offered his head. Once Ganesha received his new head, he gained the power, memory, and greatness of an elephant. Like Ganesha, we are the product of our life experiences. And no matter how challenging or painful these experiences might be, this is where our greatness often comes from.

LOVE YOUR BODY TO
LOVE YOUR MIND

Sometimes we think of the mind as being greater than the body—our analytical thought process as being somehow more important than the container that houses the mind and makes thinking possible. But the mind and the body support each other. Without one, the other can't exist. They are an inseparable pair. So embrace the body in order to embrace the mind. Thank your body for housing your brain, and for feeding and sustaining it. Love your body and mind as one.

YOUR WORDS CREATE YOUR WORLD

Words and speech can shape your days and your relationships. Today, before you speak or write a message, ask yourself what you really want to convey and if you are ready to convey it in the best way possible. Your words carry power, and used with care, that power can be an uplifting force of good. Used carelessly or vengefully, your words can become forces of destructive power. Today, try to choose your words with care, empowering yourself and the people around you.

YOGA IS:
YOUR LIFE

What happens on our yoga mat parallels what happens off our yoga mat. We encounter our struggles as well as our triumphs. We work out complicated problems, whether they are physical challenges or challenges related to our limitations and fears. We often experience a wide range of emotions during our yoga practice, just as we do in our daily lives. Every yoga practice session has a beginning, middle, and end, much like the rise and fall of a day. Throughout each session, and throughout each day, our experience can be delightful or tough, easy or difficult, frustrating or satisfying. When we can take the lessons we learn on our mats into our everyday lives, our lives become richer. We develop greater insights into the way we live. Yoga is your life.

YOU HAVE THE POWER TO OPEN YOUR HEART

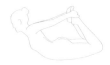

BOW POSE
DANURASANA (dah-nur-AH-sah-nah)

To open your heart and move through the world in an open-hearted way, you need to trust and feel secure in your own personal power to recognize that you have the ability to support yourself in body, mind, and heart. *Danurasana*, the Sanskrit name for Bow Pose, is the embodiment of this truth, demonstrating that when you trust your body to support you, it can lift you up. With your belly on the ground and your knees bent, reach back to take hold of your feet. Pressing your feet back into your hands, your chest lifts, opening your heart.

MANAGING
SADNESS

How can we manage sadness? First, you need to acknowledge it, to feel it within yourself. You need to accept that you are feeling something deeply, and that you cannot entirely control it. Notice what the sadness is doing to your body. Make shifts and changes in the positioning of your body by getting on your mat and moving through some yoga poses to see whether you can shift or change your physical experience of the sadness. Enter into conversation with the sadness. Excavate its origins to see if it is an isolated sadness or if it is something more deeply rooted. And then, remind yourself that this sadness—like all emotions—is temporary. It can and will pass.

END YOUR DAY WITH GRATITUDE

Today, try ending your day with a gratitude practice. Before you go to sleep, contemplate the challenges and obstacles you may have encountered, and what positive or life-affirming things may have happened to you. Ask yourself: *What went well today? What did I learn?* And if your day was challenging, ask yourself: *What do I have in my life right now for which I feel grateful?* The feeling of gratitude can shift the energy of your mind and body. The more you focus on gratitude, the more you can feel it in your mind and heart. As you conclude your day with this practice, welcome the feelings of grace and balance that emerge from the experience of gratitude.

MAKE YOUR DAY INTO MOVING MEDITATION

Today, keep your eyes open and your senses engaged, but try to move through your day with a gentle sense of direction and a commitment to staying calm, peaceful, and nonreactive. To maintain this, keep your breath steady, using it as a personal reference point. Notice whether your breath becomes rapid or agitated, and if it does, slow it down again. Imagine that your breath surrounds you, creating a private, contemplative space for you, like a protective but porous curtain between you and the world. Notice if this practice helps you find a balance between inviting the world in and maintaining your personal sense of self. Today, try to make your entire day into moving meditation.

YOUR BELLY IS A SOURCE OF INTUITION

Pay attention to what your belly tells you—it can be a source of intuition. Our bellies are sensitive, reacting not only to what we eat, but also to our emotional state. When we are nervous or anxious, our bellies often feel upset or knotted up. When we are excited about something, we may experience a fluttery feeling in our bellies. If we pay attention to these sensations, they can reveal how we feel about something before we have even consciously thought about it. Listen to what your belly is telling you for greater awareness of your emotional state and deeper insight into your thoughts and feelings.

THE MYTH OF BRAHMA AND SARASWATI CREATING THE WORLD

Brahma, the god of creation, was in the midst of forming the world. He had created mountains, oceans, and forests, and had brought all things and people into existence. At a certain point, he became overwhelmed by his creative output. Looking around, he saw chaos. He couldn't fathom how to begin organizing all that he had created. Immobilized by indecision, he closed his eyes and turned his focus inward. From the power of Brahma's inner focus and his desire for order, a fully formed being emerged from his mouth. Brahma had created Saraswati, goddess of wisdom and of the arts. Dressed in an immaculate white sari and holding a musical instrument, Saraswati looked around at everything that Brahma had produced and began to organize it. This myth shows us that creativity and order go hand and hand. Like Brahma, we must dynamically bring our thoughts and ideas into the world, and then, like Saraswati, we must begin to organize what we have created in order to fashion it into a life we love.

DEALING WITH FEELING OVERWHELMED

When you feel inundated with commitments, responsibilities, and work obligations, pause for a moment. The people who can't find the time for a yoga practice or for meditation are usually the ones who need it most. To sort through the experience of feeling overwhelmed, first try to recall what it feels like to have clarity, order, and calm. Try countering any overwrought energy with the energy of peace and centeredness. Take ten minutes to move your body through some yoga poses. Or take ten minutes to meditate. Or take ten minutes to simply close your eyes and focus on your breath. In the end, you will be better equipped to move forward calmly and get things done.

RELEASE REGRET TO FREE YOURSELF

When we allow our minds to dwell in the place of would have-could have-should have, we restrict our lives. We imprison ourselves in a web of rigid self-criticism that blinds us to our gifts and hinders our abilities to make choices and create change. Today, instead of living in a mindset of regret, try to look at where you are in the moment, and appreciate what you have learned. When a regret takes hold of you, say to yourself, *I release you as I move forward.*

MEDITATE ON THE SPACE BETWEEN THE BREATHS TO FIND PEACE

Take a deep breath. At the top of the inhale, pause for a moment. In that space just before the exhale, there is a quiet, a calmness in which everything seems peaceful and suspended. Now exhale and find a similar pause at the bottom of the breath. Again, there is a calm, a waiting, a moment just before the movement and power of the inhale begins again. This hovering place is referred to as the space between the breaths. When we direct our attention to the space between the breaths, we begin to create a sense of calm attentiveness that can last throughout our day. This is a meditation that you can practice anytime and anywhere.

WEAVE YOUR PRACTICE
THROUGHOUT YOUR DAY

One of the most meaningful things we can do as
yogis is to expand our practice from our mats out
into our lives. Think of the things we learn on our
mats: strength, tenacity, inquisitiveness, openness,
spaciousness. All of these things can be put into
action as we move through our day. Ask yourself:
*What do all of these concepts mean in my daily
life?* And, *How can I take what I learn about myself
while moving my body on my mat and apply it
to the way I think about myself and interact with
others?* Today, try weaving your yoga practice
throughout your day.

SET AN INTENTION
FOR YOUR DAY

Sankalpa Mudra (sahng-kahl-pah MOO-drah)
Mudra of Intention

What do you commit to today? What is your
intention? *Sankalpa Mudra* is a yogic hand gesture
asserting your connection to your greatest intentions, and to your heart's desire. When you sit, left
hand resting palm up on your right thigh, right palm
resting on top of the left, you hold your intention
in your hands, your body, and your consciousness.
When you make this external sign of your commitment to your goal or purpose, you deepen your
commitment. Today, form *Sankalpa Mudra* with
your hands and set an intention for your day.

ACCEPTING
WHAT IS

Much of our discontent emerges from feelings of resentment, that life is unfair, or that we somehow don't have what we need. We waste our energy focusing on how we think things should be, on how we may have arrived at a place of discontent, on the mistakes we made, or on the ways in which people may have mistreated us. We may feel that we have suffered immense personal challenges or injustices. To have peace of mind and to live satisfying lives, we can try to accept where we are and who we are. We can try to accept what is.

WHO DO YOU WANT TO BE IN THE WORLD?

Who do you want to be in the world? Ask yourself this question first thing in the morning and as you move through your day, letting your answer direct and support your actions. Do you want to be kind and patient? Let kindness and patience inform your interactions with even the most challenging people. Do you want to be courageous? Let courage override your fear, regardless of the situation. Do you want to be a good listener? Then pause, soften, and open to what others are saying. Asking yourself this question each day is like making a promise to be your best self.

LIVE WITH HOPE, NOT WITH EXPECTATION

We hope for certain events and outcomes in our lives, but we cannot control whether they happen. When we begin to expect certain outcomes, we set ourselves up for frustration and disappointment. Hope is important in that it inspires us, making us engage and invest in our lives. When we live with hope, the future opens up because hope offers possibility. When we live with expectation, the future closes down because expectation offers either success or failure. Look at your goals today, noting whether they are hopes and dreams you are working for or simply expectations. See if you can release the expectations, and instead, enjoy the sense of possibility.

YOU POSSESS ELEGANCE AND POWER

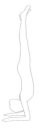

**FEATHERED PEACOCK POSE OR FOREARM
STAND POSE**
PINCHA MAYURASANA
(pin-cha mah-yoo-RAH-sah-nah)

The beauty of a peacock is in the sudden unfolding of its tail—in the surprise that such beauty was contained so discretely. When you balance on your forearms reaching your legs to the sky in *Pincha Mayurasana*, the Sanskrit name for Feathered Peacock Pose, or Forearm Stand Pose, your body mimics the upward thrust of a peacock's tail just before it opens. The beauty of the tail is displayed in the elegance of your balance and the magnificence of holding yourself upside down in such a challenging pose. Practice *Pincha Mayurasana* to demonstrate your outer elegance and your inner power.

SEE YOUR BODY AS A GIFT

We experience the world through our bodies. Our senses of sight, sound, smell, taste, and touch not only inform us about our surroundings, but they can also be sources of delight. They enable us to take pleasure in nature or in art, to enjoy a delicious meal, or to move our bodies through running, yoga, or an embrace. We often take our bodies for granted, focusing on their size or shape, and finding flaws. But our bodies enable us to be present in the world, so they are worthy of appreciation and self-care. Choose to see your body as a gift and treat it with love.

YOUR FLAWS ARE
YOUR BEAUTY

Your particularities are uniquely yours. You are an
amalgamation of all your habits, gifts, and flaws.
So embrace them. The thing that makes you feel
different or less than perfect is often what makes
you unique or special. Your particularities and
quirks have helped make you who you are right now.
And there is nothing wrong with you. What you see
as a flaw is a contribution to your individuality. So
own it. Embrace it. Your flaws are your beauty.

I BOW TO THE DIVINITY IN MYSELF AND IN ALL THINGS

Om Namah Shivaya
(ohm nah-mah shi-VAY-yah)

In yoga mythology, the god Shiva represents everything that exists, the entire universe, all of creation. This is both beautiful and awe-inspiring. We are a part of this divine universe, so when we chant *Om Namah Shivaya*, we are chanting to the beauty, wonder, and mystery of being alive. *Om* evokes everything that exists. *Namah* means that we bow down, we honor. And *Shivaya* is how we sing Shiva's name in the mantra. When we chant, we honor the divinity within ourselves. We are not separate from the divine; we are its manifestation. To that, we bow down in wonder and awe.

CONNECT WITHIN TO CONNECT WITH THE WORLD

When you are settled and connected within yourself, you are less easily shaken by external events. If your inner world is intact, your outer world is more easily managed. When we are ungrounded or anxious, we are more easily disrupted by the circumstances around us. This is why we do yoga. This is why we meditate. These practices offer us inner peace. They ground us. They create a strength that makes us more resilient in our interactions. Connect within to connect with the world.

BUILD A HEALTHY RELATIONSHIP WITH YOUR THOUGHTS

Spend the day observing your thought patterns, noticing where your thoughts wander and the ways in which you talk to yourself. If you can, take some time to journal about this at the end of the day, noting your tendencies and patterns. Did you tend to compliment yourself or criticize yourself? Did you obsess over past events, over things you can't change, or were you focused on enjoying the moment and looking toward the future? Try to keep this in mind moving forward, so when you catch yourself falling into negative thought patterns, you can more easily recognize them and choose to shift them, building a healthier relationship with your thoughts.

MANTRA
MEDITATION

Today, meditate on a sentence or phrase, making it into your daily mantra. There are an infinite number of Sanskrit mantras, but you can use the same technique of repetition using your own content. You can repeat a line from a poem, a saying that resonates with you, or a mantra of your own invention. Whether you are sitting for meditation, commuting to work, or taking a break in a crowded place, return to your mantra throughout your day and repeat it either silently or out loud, depending on where you are. Using a mantra for meditation is a great way to keep your mind focused, to calm yourself, and to connect with something that is meaningful to you.

YOUR LOVE IS LIMITLESS

No matter how many people, places, and things you love, and how intensely you love them, you will always have more love. Think of your love as being like the ocean: There are places where it is shallow and places where it is deep. There are areas that are tranquil and areas of turbulence. But no matter how many different experiences you have of love, your love is vast and unlimited like the ocean. Your love cannot be dispersed or diluted no matter how many times you love or how many people, places, and things you love. You are never without love for a moment of your life because your love is limitless.

SINUOUS STRENGTH

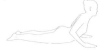

COBRA POSE

BHUJANGASANA (boo-jan-GAH-sah-nah)

Resting the fronts of your legs on the ground, curl your torso up and back like a cobra raising its head for *Bhujangasana*, the Sanskrit word for Cobra Pose. Look around, gliding your torso side to side, warming up your back, your spine, and your waist. You can begin curling into a gentle, supported lift, like a baby cobra, then reach your heart forward, arching into more of a backbend, like a bigger cobra rising to strike. Like a cobra, your movement is graceful and sinuous yet powerful. Relaxed but alert, like the cobra, you are poised for action.

OFFERING
COMFORT

Imagine: A friend comes to you, upset about something. You offer to listen to their frustration, creating a safe place for them to release and relax. Perhaps they need a hug. Perhaps they simply need to be heard. You are offering them comfort. Odds are, they don't want or need for you to tell them what to do, although that is often our inclination. Offering comfort to someone involves less effort than you may imagine. It often requires just offering them a safe place to unwind.

HONOR YOUR
DREAMS

To achieve your dreams, begin by honoring them.
To honor your dreams, treat them like your babies,
serving them, nurturing them, feeding them, and
making sure they thrive. Organize your life in a way
that supports your creative vision and aspirations
for your future. Resist giving in to the doubts that
others may have about your dreams. When you
have a moment of self-doubt, remember that you
must sometimes even protect your dreams from
yourself. Make caring for your dreams a daily practice. Ask yourself: *What have I done to honor my
dreams today?*

THE MYTH OF BABY KRISHNA, MUD PIES, AND THE UNIVERSE

One day, back when the god Krishna was a baby, he was playing in the yard with the neighbor's son, happily making sand castles and mud pies. Krishna's mother, Yashoda, who was keeping an eye on the boys, suddenly saw Krishna cramming mud into his mouth. She rushed over to him, scolded him, and grabbed his face to clean it. As she peered into his mouth, Krishna mischievously revealed the entire universe within it. Overcome by what she saw, Yashoda fainted. Krishna was immediately remorseful. He called to Maya, the goddess of illusion, and implored her to conceal what he had revealed. When Yashoda recovered, she had forgotten what she had seen. This myth shows us how perceiving the world in one small glimpse or experience at a time enables us to appreciate it. Be fully present in each small moment, and the universe will reveal itself slowly and beautifully.

ABUNDANCE OFFERS CHOICE

The Sanskrit word *shri* (shree) means that which is abundant, beautiful, and auspicious. Interestingly, *shri* also means precise and selective. These two different meanings might seem contradictory, but abundance and selectivity actually go hand in hand. To be selective and make wise choices, we must approach our selections with a mindset of abundance, rather than mistakenly believing that only a few options are available to us. In reality, a multitude of options is always available to us. We can adopt a mindset of abundance by being open to new ideas and to the opinions of others. With more ideas and options in our lives, we are in a state of abundance. We can make wiser and more accurate decisions about what we want and about how to achieve our goals. Abundance offers us choice in our lives.

PRACTICE MINDFULNESS IN YOUR LIFE

Being mindful means bringing awareness and intentionality to your ways of thinking, speaking, and acting in the world. Mindfulness is something you can practice on a regular basis. Today, the minute you notice yourself making a snap judgment about something, pause for a moment. Notice what your mind is doing with the situation. Notice, for example, whether you are indulging in self-criticism or negativity toward others, and if you are, stop yourself in the act. Try to identify what individual or circumstance triggered this shift, and decide to disengage with that negative energy. To practice mindfulness, invite your mind to observe its patterns so you can change them if needed. In the process, a kinder, more thoughtful you may emerge. You begin to move through your daily life with an awareness of your behavior, which ultimately can offer you a more settled mind and heart.

YOGA IS:
ARTISTRY

Practicing yoga is creative. You arrange your body in a series of yoga poses, shifting and adjusting within each pose to create alignment. Each pose offers a particular exploration and consequent experience of your body and yourself. That experience may be stability, exuberance, energy, inquisitiveness, peace, or a combination of several of these qualities, similar to the way in which an artwork is composed of many elements coming together to form a surprising whole. By choosing which poses to take, sequencing them, and engaging with them in a mindful way, you enter into a creative dialogue with your yoga practice, in which the finished experience is greater than the sum of its parts. Your practice is a symphony, a painting, a dance. Yoga is artistry.

LIKE NATURE, YOU EBB AND FLOW

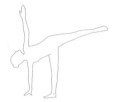

HALF MOON POSE
ARDHA CHANDRASANA
(ar-dah chan-DRAH-sah-nah)

Rise up into *Ardha Chandrasana*, the Sanskrit name
for Half Moon Pose. Balancing on one foot and on
the fingertips of one hand, reach one arm toward the
sky and root the other to the ground. You become
the landscape: the earth, the moon and stars,
and everything that moves among them. Opening
sideways, your entire body is visible from one angle,
but from another, you only see a portion of your
body. Like the moon, you have times when you are
expansive and times when you are smaller and more
discrete. Like nature, you ebb and flow. Embrace the
process.

ACCESS
JOY

There are so many ways we can access joy. Begin by finding something that generates the feeling of joy within you. This could be a small meaningful gift someone has given you or it could be something from nature. Joy can reside in an activity you love, something you read, or a piece of music. Joy can reside in the smallest thing. When you feel yourself in need of joy, turn to one of these sources. Listen to that song, do a Downward-Facing Dog Pose, draw a picture, go for a walk—hold that object in your hands or in your heart to remind yourself of the sensation of joy. You always have access to joy.

THE IMPORTANCE
OF RITUAL

Rituals create meaning. They are a way of honoring the people in our lives, the things we love, and our belief systems. An action, consciously taken and repeated, gathers meaning by ritually focusing our attention on whatever it is that we are honoring. Think of some everyday rituals, from giving thanks at the beginning of a meal to lighting a candle in remembrance of someone we love or miss. A ritual can take the form of morning meditation or yoga practice. Over time, these rituals accumulate power through the act of their repetition. They give meaning and structure to our lives.

BE CONSISTENT TO BE TRUE TO YOURSELF

Your behavior is the expression of your thoughts and beliefs. Every action you take is an illustration of your values. Ask yourself: *Is the way I behave in the world true to my values, my thinking, and my belief system? Are my acts consistent with my words?* To be true to yourself, your internal thinking and your external behavior must be in an ongoing relationship of aligning and realigning. Even though we change and the world around us changes, we can be consistent in our behavior, thereby demonstrating our integrity.

MEDITATE ON LOVE

When you think of love, what comes to mind? If it is a person or a thing, look a little more closely, noticing the particular qualities that inspire your love. If thinking about love generates a sensation within you, examine that, noticing where you might find that impulse in your body and then what type of a sensation it is. Next, see if you can connect with an overall feeling of love, of experiencing the emotion in your own body and mind apart from any specific love object. In this way, you begin to tap into a more universal concept and experience of love. Know that this love is always available to you. Let this be your meditation today.

YOUR BODY
IS BEAUTIFUL

From where you are sitting, take a look at your
body. First, take note of its overall form. Then,
notice your body's distinctive characteristics,
what marks it as uniquely yours. Appreciate its
similarities to other people's bodies, which serve
as reminders of your deep connectivity to every
other human being. Then take delight in your physical uniqueness, recognizing the individuality of your
particular beauty. Your own personal version of
beauty is something to be treasured. Always remind
yourself that your body is beautiful exactly as it is.

THE MYTH OF LAKSHMI AND THE GARLAND OF FLOWERS

A sage approached Indra, the great ancient king of the gods, and offered him a garland of flowers. Distractedly, Indra pushed the garland to the side without thanking him. Lakshmi, goddess of beauty and abundance, was horrified at Indra's ungrateful behavior and his rejection of the beautiful garland. She dove into the ocean of consciousness, taking all beauty and abundance with her. The gods, reeling from the absence of Lakshmi and her virtues, called to Lakshmi's beloved Vishnu, the great sustainer of life, hoping that his love could draw her back into the world so that it would be filled with beauty and richness again. Vishnu convinced the gods to join forces with the powerful demons, so together they could vigorously churn the ocean and find her. After days of churning, their efforts worked. Lakshmi arose from the ocean, standing on a lotus blossom, and ushered beauty back into the world. Lakshmi's action reminds us that beauty should never be taken for granted. May we always receive beauty with gratitude.

BREATHE AND EMBRACE YOUR HEART

Wherever you are right now, take a deep breath. Feel your lungs swelling against your rib cage, and your ribs expanding and lifting. Your lungs are expanding within as well, swelling around your heart. Consider this: With every inhale, your body embraces your body. Your lungs embrace your heart. No matter where you are or what you are experiencing at any given moment, as you breathe, you are in a state of constant self-embrace.

YOGA OFFERS AN OPPORTUNITY TO EXPERIENCE YOURSELF

Every time you set foot on your mat, you are opening to a new experience of yourself. Sometimes it is a delight to practice and other times it is hard to motivate yourself. When you are feeling this hesitancy or procrastination, remind yourself that your yoga practice is not an obligation. It is an opportunity to explore and open your body. Every day's practice is different, and your response to your practice each day may be different as well, depending on the season, your mood, and the type of practice you do. Your yoga practice is an opportunity to experience yourself in a new way every day.

ON WAKING UP

In that first moment of awareness when you awaken, you are in a different type of consciousness. You are not entirely awake, yet you are no longer asleep. You are in a quiet place, a place of pause, that is somewhere in between. One morning, upon waking, see if you can stay in that place of quiet, not falling back to sleep yet not rushing forward into your day. Stay in that pause, in that open state between sleep and alertness, allowing your brain to hover in the transition between the sleeping and waking worlds. Appreciate the experience of living in these two worlds simultaneously. Remind yourself that there are always more corners of our consciousness to explore.

THE PELVIS HOLDS CREATIVE POWER

The pelvis is generative, powerful, and often mysterious to us. When we begin a yoga practice, we become more acutely aware of the complexity of the muscles weaving in and around our pelvis, the connection of the spine, and the movement of the hips. Our pelvis forms a vessel holding both procreative power and desire. When we sit for meditation, drawing the energy of the breath all the way down to this center, we feel grounded and inwardly focused. We begin to access our earthy creative impulses. The pelvis is the center of our creative power.

BE THE
CHANGE

A quote sometimes attributed to the great advocate of peaceful resistance, Mahatma Gandhi, is: "Be the change you wish to see in the world." This is a valuable invitation to us. To be the change, begin with awareness and move toward action. Being the change involves knowledge of your core values and beliefs. Then ask yourself: *How can I give my values shape and form in the world?* Choose to speak your mind, standing up for what you believe to be right and against injustices that you see. Check to make sure that your actions illustrate your words. Being the change is about alignment and integrity. Do the inner work of cultivating attentiveness and awareness to do the outer work of taking action and being a force for good in the world.

EXPAND YOUR AWARENESS

Padma Mudra (pahd-mah MOO-drah)
Lotus Mudra

Connect the base of your palms in front of your heart, flaring out your fingers as if you were holding a ball between your hands. Your palms and the rest of your fingers form what looks like an open vessel or blossoming flower. This hand gesture is *Padma Mudra. Padma* is the Sanskrit word for lotus. The lotus represents consciousness, its plentiful petals unfolding one by one, demonstrating how your awareness of yourself and of the universe can expand endlessly. Deities are often depicted sitting or standing on lotus blossoms, indicating different experiences you can have when you open to receive what the universe is offering you.

LET
IT GO

Let it go. How important is it really, anyway? Is
it life or death? Or is it something that has been
fixed in your mind for so long that you simply can't
release it? Once you truly let something go, you
free yourself from the tyranny of a thought or of a
habit. You can now choose a different way of thinking or being, and more importantly, you open up
to receive a greater range of thoughts and experiences. Your act of release unlocks the world's
abundance and welcomes it into your life. Simply
soften, release, and receive.

YOGA IS:
INQUIRY

Our yoga practice offers us a wide range of experiences, from curiosity and delight to intensity and strength. When we step onto our mats to practice, we do not know exactly what we will experience. Yoga is not an exact science. It invites us to explore and experience, and offers the possibility of insight and transformation. By inviting us to live in this place of possibility, yoga shows us that we have the capacity to feel deeply and to explore endlessly. Yoga shows us that every practice is an inquiry into ourselves, inviting us to personal understandings and a larger, richer universe.

BALANCE YOUR HEAD
AND YOUR HEART

Your heart and your head are not always in agreement with each other. Sometimes your heart may powerfully desire something that your head knows is not good for you. At other times, your head may take over excessively, filling you with mental chatter and blocking out the voice of your heart. The trick is to balance your head and heart as much as possible so that you hear both. Today, take a moment to ask yourself these two questions: *What is my heart's desire right now? What is my mind telling me about this?* Then, see if you can join the wisdom of your mind and heart, finding some sort of middle ground between what you desire and what you think you should or should not desire in order to gain perspective and to find balance.

USE YOUR STRENGTH
BUT STAY GROUNDED

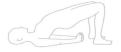

BRIDGE POSE
SETU BANDHA SARVANGASANA (say-too bahn-dah
sar-VAN-GAH-sah-nah)

Setu Banda Sarvangasana, the Sanskrit name for
Bridge Pose, takes a moderate amount of strength
but feels supportive and grounding. The pose asks
you to arrange your body in the same way that a
bridge is held together: arching up with tensile
strength while connecting solidly to the ground
at both ends. Supporting yourself on your head,
shoulders, and the soles of your feet, reach your
body upward to create a bridge shape. Because of
the support of your shoulders and head at one end
and your feet at the other end, your chest, pelvis,
and thighs can arch upward gracefully, delineating
the curved shape of a bridge while safely opening the front of your body and offering stability
through structure.

DISCOVER A UNIVERSE IN EVERY SMALL OBJECT

In this moment, and throughout the day, look around and notice the small objects in your environment. If you are outdoors, you might gaze upon a leaf or a blade of grass. If you are at home, it could be anything from a glass of water to a cherished keepsake. Focus on this chosen object for a few minutes, noticing its shape, color, and texture. Where did it come from? How did it come to be in your personal world? The more intensely we focus, the more expansive an object becomes, until we see that it contains a whole universe. We can discover a universe in anything and everything. Then, when we turn our attention back out into the greater world, we have a sense of the vastness of everything around us. Our world becomes richer.

EMBRACE YOUR MULTIFACETED SELF

You reveal different aspects of your personality when you are with different people. Who you are while in the company of a friend or family member is different from who you are with a lover, a colleague, or an acquaintance. Today, notice which of your qualities are brought out by the different people around you. You may have a patient or nurturing self that interacts with a child, a dynamic self for professional interactions, a romantic and sensual self for your beloved. You are vast and complex. Embrace your multifaceted self today.

MAY I ALWAYS DO THE RIGHT THING

Shri Ram Jai Ram Jai Jai Ram
(shree rahm jay rahm jay jay rahm)

Ram, whose name appears in this mantra, is the ultimate god of *dharma*, which can be defined as righteousness, truth, and duty. In yoga mythology, Ram upholds laws and virtue. When we wish to do the right thing no matter how challenging and difficult it may be, we can chant his mantra. *Shri* means auspicious or life-affirming, and *Jai* is an exclamation of honoring and victory. When we chant *Shri Ram Jai Ram Jai Jai Ram*, we are saying, "Let my actions and behavior be exemplary. May I uphold truth, and may I maintain harmony through order and structure in my life."

YOU ARE
NEVER ALONE

You are intimately and intricately connected to the
entire world. When any of us feels alone, it is often
because of insecurity, fear, or anxiety. But we all
share these emotions. When you are lonely, remind
yourself that you are connected to everything that
lives. We all breathe the same air. We all walk on the
same earth. We share similar hopes, fears, dreams,
and passions. We exist in similar bodies and are
subjected to the same conditions of being human.
We are deeply and inseparably linked. Today,
remember that you are woven into the fabric of
this interconnectivity. You are never alone.

SET GOALS BUT STAY FLEXIBLE

Personal achievement starts with identifying what you want, setting goals, then constructing a plan and mapping out the steps to achieve your objectives. As you do this, recognize that goals shift with circumstances, so try not to be so rigid that you become stuck when things don't turn out exactly as planned. Be flexible and open. Think of what it's like to hold your body in a yoga pose. If you are completely rigid, someone can easily tip you over, but if you are not locked in place, you can move, bend, and adapt. Your goals are like your pose: your adaptability is key in each. So, as you move forward in your life, be ready to shift, change, and grow into a new place.

CULTIVATE PEACE IN YOUR DAILY LIFE

To feel peaceful, try to cultivate peace in your life on a daily basis. Cultivating peace involves spending more time engaging in activities that foster this feeling within you, whether it is getting out in nature, going for a walk in the city, or sitting to meditate. Surround yourself with people who share your vision and support your dreams, so you engage in harmonious conversation and interaction. Arrange your home in a way that feels inviting and restful. Embrace each aspect of your life that nurtures your inner calm and creates an inner and outer tranquility in your life.

LOVING KINDNESS MEDITATION

Loving kindness meditation can generate kindness, compassion, and feelings of love toward ourselves and others. To begin a loving kindness meditation practice, close your eyes and offer love, acceptance, and compassion to yourself, inwardly saying words such as: *May I be happy, healthy, loved, and at peace.* Let the meaning of these words sink in, feeling the loving kindness that you are offering to yourself. Then inwardly, to a friend or loved one, say: *May you be happy, healthy, loved, and at peace.* Next, inwardly offer the words to an acquaintance, then to someone whom you may find challenging or difficult. Finally, offer the words to all of these people and all other beings you can imagine, so you create a vast field of loving kindness within yourself. When you are ready, gently open your eyes.

WHAT DO YOU VALUE? GIVE IT LIFE IN THE WORLD

Ask yourself: *What are the things I truly love and value?* What immediately comes to mind may be a person, a place, a cause, or an object. Identify these as your values and let them guide your actions. Consider how they can shape your thinking and your life choices. Your actions are demonstrations of your point of view, so notice what your actions tell you about whether they are aligned with your values. Whatever you value, express it in your everyday life through your words and your actions. Give your values life by drawing what resides in your heart out into the world.

BALANCE YOUR BODY TO FIND EASE IN YOUR HEART

CRANE POSE
BAKASANA (ba-KAH-sah-nah)

When we talk about creating balance in our lives, we are often looking for an experience of ease and calm. Sometimes balance seems elusive, but when we find it in one aspect of our lives, we can often bring it into other parts as well. *Bakasana* is the Sanskrit word for Crane Pose. When we connect our hands firmly to the ground, balance our bent knees on the back of our upper arms, and rise into *Bakasana*, our spirits also lift and we begin to experience that sense of ease. The more balanced we are in our bodies, the more our minds and hearts can rise and open.

EMPATHY HELPS US UNDERSTAND OTHERS

We can more truly understand others if we become attentive to their emotions, feelings, and experiences. We gain wisdom by comparing their experiences with our own, seeing our commonalities and our differences, and experiencing what they may feel. Through empathy, we begin to see that many of us want the same things in life: love, happiness, success, adventure, respect, and peace. Sometimes, we struggle to understand another person's behavior, especially when it appears to be highly emotional, confrontational, or feels hurtful to us. When this happens, think: *What could be at the root of these feelings or this behavior?* And if we really think about it, we may discover that the root will probably be the wish for something that we also want out of life. From this understanding, compassion can grow.

HONOR YOUR EXPERIENCES

Our experiences, no matter how complex or simple, are of value. We are the cumulative result of our experiences and how we have processed them. The people and events of our lives have taught us, surprised us, embarrassed us, and delighted us. What we have done and whom we have loved and not loved have all contributed to who we are now. Today, think about your life as a story, and who the major characters and events might be. Your life story is as rich as any story you might read. Your experiences create the narrative of your life. Honor your experiences.

THE MYTH OF PARVATI AND SHIVA'S DICE GAME

The goddess Parvati loved to play a dice game with her husband, the god Shiva. Each time they played, the game began with teasing, then progressed to fierce competition, trickery, and cheating. At the end of each game, Parvati would distract Shiva with her beauty, win the game, and then Shiva would storm off to meditate in the mountains. After a while, they would miss each other, and Shiva would finally return to their home, where the game would begin again. Life is filled with harmony and conflict, passion and strife. The questions you must ask yourself are: *How deeply and fully do I want to experience life? Am I willing to aim high in my ambitions with the possibility of failure? Am I willing to get my heart broken?* If you hold back, you will be living a half-life, constrained by fear and self-imposed limitations. Take the risk. Choose to engage fully in life with all of its challenges.

ON YOGA AND INTUITION

Our yoga practice can make us more conscious of our environment and more sensitive to the people around us. This shift may foster a stronger connection to our intuition. Our intuition can increase our awareness of other people's feelings and thoughts, enhancing our ability to connect to them. We may notice how people respond to us more acutely, or we may sense when something is either very wrong or very right in a particular situation. Because yoga develops our awareness of our bodies, it often helps us develop a corresponding awareness that extends beyond our physical selves and into our mental, emotional, and intuitive lives.

THANK PEOPLE IN YOUR LIFE TODAY

How often do you feel thankful but don't find the words to express your feelings? How often do you feel grateful to someone but think that what you have to offer in the way of thanks is insufficient? Release that thinking and take action today by expressing your gratitude to them. Any sincere expression of thanks is meaningful. It doesn't need to be original or grandiose. Letting people know how you feel is what counts. Today, say thank you to the people who have helped, inspired, and loved you. Let them know you are grateful. Draw it out of your heart and into the world.

YOGA IS:
GRACE

Grace is a quality that means slightly different things to different people, so it is difficult to define. To some of us, grace feels like we are being held by something greater than ourselves. To others, it feels like things in our lives are falling perfectly into place. To still others, it feels as if we are existing in a state of harmony with the world. Whatever grace may feel like to you, consider this: grace is within. You don't need to beg for it or think that it is something outside of yourself. Grace is something you already possess. It is something tucked within you that you can call on when you need it. Yoga's ability to align body, heart, and mind offers us the experience of grace. This deep connectivity offered by yoga is grace itself.

LOOK
WITHIN

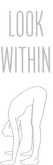

STANDING FORWARD BEND POSE
UTTANASANA (OO-tah-NAS-sah-nah)

Uttanasana, the Sanskrit name for Standing Forward Bend, invites you to stand, fold your torso
over your legs, and allow your upper body to hang
toward the ground. With your head facing your
legs, you are in a position to look within. For some,
this pose is easy and relaxing, while for others it is
demanding. Looking within yourself requires a combination of effort and surrender. It's a process in
which you examine your life and recognize what you
can and cannot change. However deeply you are
able to experience this pose—whether your spine
is curved or straight, whether your hands touch
the ground or not—the pose lends itself to a hybrid
experience of effort and ease, mirroring your own
process of introspection.

CALMING
ANXIETY

What happens to you when you become anxious?
Try to remember a moment of great anxiety in your
life and recall what the experience was like. Some
common physical symptoms are a racing heart,
sweating or feeling faint, or developing a headache
or backache. Some people have difficulty speaking. The common thread is how our emotional or
mental state affects our physical being. When we
can read our physical symptoms, we can address
anxiety when it arises. We can deepen our breath,
shift or stretch our bodies, or drink a glass of water,
reminding ourselves that this particular experience
will pass. In this way, we can often calm the symptoms of anxiety and quiet our hearts.

GETTING OUT OF OUR OWN WAY

Sometimes we make things more complicated than we need to. We explain to our friends that we can't do this because of that, or we have countless reasons why we can't get around to making that phone call, having that conversation, or making that life change. The excuses pile up, cluttering the space of possibility until the solutions feel stuck beneath them. By practicing awareness, we can recognize what we are doing and try to stop. We can ask ourselves, *What do I really want?* And when the answer comes, we can find the simplest and most direct manner of achieving it. Sometimes the complications are self-created and we have the power to change, to simplify, and to move forward.

MEDITATE IN A CROWD

Meditation is commonly perceived to be an activity that is performed alone in a quiet place without disruptions. Today, expand your own experience of meditation by practicing in a crowd of people. Find a shared public space. Begin by softening your gaze and turning your attention within. Releasing any resistance to the sounds that surround you, invite them in as keys that can unlock your meditation. Or, think of these sounds as food to feed your meditation so that you feel nourished by your environment. Each sound, like a taste of the world, is an opportunity to expand your meditation from a closed, singular experience to a vast, expansive one.

YOUR RIB CAGE IS THE GUARDIAN OF YOUR LUNGS AND HEART

Consider how your ribs form a graceful fence around your heart, lungs, and other organs. Your rib cage, made of bone and cartilage, is strong and durable yet also supple and resilient. It rises and falls with your breath, and bends and gives while protecting. Hold your hands in front of you. Spread your fingers and connect the base of your palms and the tips of your curved fingers as if you were gently holding an invisible heart. This is what your ribs do inside your body. Powerful but delicate, strong but elegant, your ribs structure your torso, embrace your organs, and pulse with your breath.

THE MYTH OF HANUMAN'S LEAP ACROSS THE SEA

Hanuman, the monkey deity who was devoted to the great god Ram and his beautiful goddess Sita, was on a quest to find Sita, who had been kidnapped by the terrifying multiheaded demon Ravana. Ravana had hidden Sita in his vast palace in Lanka, the kingdom across the sea, so Hanuman leapt across the water to find her. After he had flown through the air for many hours, the gods placed a mountain in his path for him to rest on, but Hanuman shoved it aside with his shoulder. Shortly after this, a giant sea snake rose out of the water to attack him. Hanuman shrank himself to the size of a bug, and, flying straight into the sea snake's mouth, escaped out one of her nostrils. Focused in his mission, Hanuman finally arrived at the shores at Lanka, where he located Sita and instigated her rescue. Like Hanuman, let your devotion guide your actions, and be undeterred in your mission.

EACH EXHALE IS AN OPPORTUNITY TO RELEASE

Each exhale is an opportunity to release something more than just the breath. We can choose to release physical tension and stress. We can rid ourselves of feelings and thoughts that are not serving us, exhaling them away, again and again. Sometimes the simple action of exhaling invites relaxation in our bodies. We can make this a practice by using the exhale to release a troubling thought or to release a knot of tension in our bodies. Throughout your day today, try using your exhale as a way of releasing a thought or physical sensation that is not serving you.

PRACTICE AND FLOURISH

Yoga flourishes through a balanced and reasonable amount of discipline. Commit to your practice. Set modest realistic goals for yourself and make the daily attainment of these goals your personal practice. Like any discipline, there will be times when your yoga practice feels deeply fulfilling and times when it feels burdensome. In the challenging times, remind yourself of why you are doing it. Practice even when you have doubt in order to create a life of yoga for yourself. A reasonable degree of discipline offers tremendous rewards.

WANTING WHAT YOU DON'T HAVE

We live in a consumer society in which we are continuously told what we need through advertisements and through comparison to the people around us. As a result, we find ourselves always wanting more. Take a minute today to notice where this impulse manifests in your life. What are you longing for that you don't have? Do you really need it? There is a big difference between what we need and what we want. We need shelter, food, health, and safety. We may want new possessions, professional success, and recognition, but we don't actually need those things. Ask yourself: *Is this something that I need? Or is it something that I want?* Evaluate your answers and allocate your resources and attention accordingly.

BECOMING SPACIOUS IN OUR BODIES, HEARTS, AND MINDS

We often hear the term spaciousness in the yoga world. It can refer to an experience of the body, the heart, the mind, or all three. When we think about spaciousness, we think of having space in which to move, to reflect, and to grow. When we move our bodies on our mats, our bodies become more open, more spacious, offering ease, relief, and maybe joy. This can create an equivalent opening in our minds and in our hearts, causing us to become more mentally and emotionally ready to receive what the world is offering. This is spaciousness, and we cultivate it through our yoga practice.

CLEAR THE WAY FOR AN ABUNDANT LIFE

Shankha Mudra (SHAN-khah MOO-drah)
Conch Shell Mudra

We all want to thrive. The *shankha*, the Sanskrit word for conch shell, is used in some cultures as a trumpet; the loud noise issuing from it is seen as clearing the space around us to make room for prosperity, fertility, and abundance. To invite these positive qualities into your own life, form *Shankha Mudra*, a hand gesture in the shape of a conch. Curl the four fingers of your right hand around your left thumb like a fist, and extend your right thumb and your left fingers so they touch at the top just above the fist. The inner fingers framed by the outer fingers will resemble the shell. Use *Shankha Mudra* to affirm abundance and prosperity in your life.

YOGA EMPOWERS US

When we move our bodies through yoga poses, we acquire a sense of control within our bodies that translates into a greater sense of control within our lives. This can be empowering, for it offers us insights into the working of our bodies and the ways in which the condition of our bodies affects our minds and our spirits. We can more readily pinpoint what we are feeling in our bodies and often what we are feeling in our hearts. Yoga also offers us the experience of bodily strength and a way of creating beauty through and with our bodies. Yoga empowers us.

CONNECT YOUR MIND AND YOUR HEART TO FIND WISDOM

We possess an intelligence of the mind and an intelligence of the heart. When we operate from only one of these places, we limit our understanding of ourselves and of the world around us. When we join our mind's analytical abilities with our heart-centered emotional selves, we become more insightful: we possess a greater way of taking in the world and understanding it. We develop wisdom. As you move through your day today, notice the balance between your mental intelligence and your emotional intelligence, and invite both to inform your thoughts and actions.

SIMPLIFY YOUR DAY BY PRIORITIZING AND LETTING GO

Today, when you feel frenzied or overwhelmed, simplify. Sometimes we try to juggle too much, which makes us feel scattered and incapable of completing anything. Pause for a moment. Ask yourself: *Which of these things do I have to do and which of these things can wait until later? And which of these things can I let go of altogether?* Simplify your day by prioritizing and letting go. Then, make a methodical plan for calmly moving forward step by step.

THE BEAUTIFUL GEOMETRY
OF YOU

TRIANGLE POSE
TRIKONASANA (tree-koh-NAH-sah-nah)

Imagine creating an origami flower by folding a sheet of paper back and forth into angles until you open one last fold to reveal the beauty of the final form. *Trikonasana*, the Sanskrit name for Triangle Pose, invites you to fold your body into a similarly beautiful form. To practice this pose, step one foot forward, and turn the toes of your back foot out to the side. Bow over your front straight leg to touch the floor outside of your foot, then open your torso to the side. Complete the pose by extending your top arm toward the sky. This final gesture opens up the body like the dramatic final fold of the origami flower. In Triangle Pose, your body becomes artfully moving geometry.

TREAT YOUR BODY LIKE A SACRED SPACE

Consider what it means to treat your body like a sacred space. What food and drink will you put into your body? What will you apply to the skin of your body? How will you dress your body? Will you treat your body with kindness, making sure it gets enough rest, grooming, and nurturing? Imagine your body as a temple: at the center of the temple is your heart, up top is your mind, and all of it is permeated with your spirit. As a temple, how should it be cared for? When you treat your body with the same reverence as you would a sacred place, your body will respond. Today, invite your eating, breathing, and moving to become a form of prayer.

LET IT
BE

Swaha
(SWA-ha)

Sometimes we need to recognize when something is blocking us in our lives, and release it. It could be a thought that doesn't serve us, a grudge, a nagging anxiety, or a situation we cannot change. To let it go, we chant the mantra *Swaha*, a Sanskrit term that means so be it, let it be, or let it burn. Letting go of habits, ideas, or relationships that no longer serve us is one of the greatest challenges we face on a daily basis, but it is an essential practice for moving forward in our lives. Take a deep breath, soften, and say: *Swaha, Swaha, Swaha.*

YOU ARE YOUR OWN GURU

The Sanskrit word *guru* (GOO-roo) means a teacher. Anything and everything can be a teacher if we let it. The blade of grass that pushes its way up through a crack in the concrete shows us about tenacity and determination. A person who guides us academically or in life teaches us facts and skills. Our friends and family are our teachers, as are strangers and acquaintances, whether or not we like the lessons they offer. As we move through our days, there are infinite lessons we can learn and an infinite number of people or things that teach us. In the end, we need to gather, sift through, and choose from these experiences in order to be our own best teachers, our own gurus.

MEDITATE ON THE INNER BODY

Today, take a moment to sit quietly and close your eyes. Draw your attention to the surface of your skin, noticing any sensations you are feeling: heat, cold, the movement of the air around you, or pressure. Then draw your attention into your body, to the fat that sits just beneath the surface of your skin: soft, insulating, and protective. Slowly shift your attention to the muscles, ligaments, and tendons of your body, feeling their tensile strength. Next, focus on the fluids and organs of your body: the blood pumping through your veins and the many intricate workings of your internal organs. Finally, draw your attention to the durable architecture of your bones and your elaborate skeletal system. Now expand your attention to your entire body at once, and simply breathe. When you are ready, ease out of the meditation, breath by breath, and then open your eyes. This meditation on the inner body can bring you a sense of wonder about the complexity of your inner world.

OFFER LOVE TO GENERATE LOVE IN THE WORLD

Deciding to offer love to another person is not about immediate reciprocity; the point is that by offering love, you are generating more love in the world, and thereby generating more love in your life. Everyone benefits. It is true that if you offer loving behavior toward others, you are more likely to receive love. But even if the love you offer is not reciprocated, you have shown yourself that you possess so much love that you are able to offer it freely. Love offered is never wasted; a surplus of love in the world could only be positive. So offer love. Generate love. Be loving. You have nothing to lose and everything to gain.

EMBRACE YOUR GREATNESS TO SEE THE GREATNESS IN OTHERS

The Sanskrit word *adhikara* (ahd-hee-KAH-rah) means one's own individual gifts, skills, and sensibility, what each human being can best offer to the world. Recognizing your *adhikara* means recognizing your own innate gifts, owning the greatness that you possess as a result of those gifts, and letting that knowledge and power guide you in the world. When you are comfortable with who you are and confident about what you have to offer, you are better able to see the greatness in others. By embracing your *adhikara*, you embrace the gifts of others as well.

THE MYTH OF GANESHA AND CHANDRA

The elephant-headed god Ganesha arrived one evening in the village where sweets had been made and left to cool. He breathed in the delicious aroma of the sweets, and tried one. As soon as he swallowed it, he could not restrain himself, and ate them all. Embarrassed, he climbed onto his mouse, Musika, to make his escape. He was so heavy that Musika stumbled, tipping over Ganesha, whose belly opened, spilling out the sweets. Ganesha heard laughter. He looked into the sky and saw Chandra, the moon god, mocking him. Frustrated, Ganesha hurled his broken tusk at Chandra, shattering him, telling him that from this point on, Chandra would wax and wane, and on the final day of his waning, he would resemble Ganesha's tusk. Both Ganesha's plight and Chandra's fate show us that when we take in the world in one small amount at a time, we are better able to savor it, and that we, too, wax and wane. We don't need to have everything all at once.

BALANCE DREAMS AND REALITY

Are you more of a realist or a dreamer? This question may seem easy to answer in one way or the other, but we are actually a combination of both. Your dreams help you develop ambitious plans and fantasies, and to feel no constraint as you imagine your future. Your realist side may build logically and rationally on what you know yourself to be capable of, using your skills and gifts. When we can balance our dreamer selves with our rational selves, we can be boundlessly creative and then apply our practicality to making our dreams into reality.

FIND THE EXPERIENCE OF PEACE BY TURNING WITHIN

The moment you start paying attention to the inner workings of your body, you begin to connect with the experience of peace. Take a moment today to try this exercise: First, close your eyes and quiet your mind and body. Feel the rise and fall of your breath. Listen to the beat of your heart, the throb of your pulse. Invite your mind to travel through your body, experiencing your most internal sensations. By cultivating this deep inner attentiveness, you move into the vast landscape of your inner body, in which resides an even deeper experience of peace.

YOGA IS:
DEVOTION

The Sanskrit word for devotion—such as the devotion we feel for our loved ones, for something we believe in, or for a cause close to our heart—is *bhakti* (BHAKH-tee). In yoga, *bhakti* practices include chanting mantras, making offerings, and other acts of reverence. These practices have the capacity to help us feel connected to others and to causes greater than ourselves. *Bhakti* can be as simple as setting an intention, devoting our daily yoga practice to someone in need, or lighting a candle in someone's memory and saying a prayer. When we engage in any form of *bhakti*, we offer our best selves to the world and welcome the peaceful-ness that often follows.

MAY YOUR OUTER FORM HONOR YOUR INNER BEAUTY

GARLAND POSE
MALASANA (mah-LAH-sah-nah)

In the yoga tradition, a mala is a string of beads or a garland of flowers. It is a blessing, a tool, an ornament, and an acknowledgment of beauty. Draping a garland of flowers over someone is a way of honoring him or her. Repeating a mantra while moving your fingers along the beads of a mala is a practice of devotion and a meditation technique. When you crouch down in *Malasana*, or Garland Pose, a squatting position with your arms resting between your knees and your palms together in prayer, your outer form—your body—honors your inner beauty. When you practice this pose, imagine yourself wrapped in garlands of flowers and lengths of prayer beads. Recognize that you are worthy of honor and offer this to yourself.

RELEASE JEALOUSY

When jealousy arises within ourselves, it is often because we feel that we have less than we deserve or we see something another person has that we feel should be ours. There are few emotions as insidious and counterproductive to our well-being as jealousy, so it benefits us to release it. Jealousy eats away at us from the inside: it is a totally self-destructive experience. So the next time jealousy arises within you, ask yourself: *Is this what I want to feel right now?* If not, treat it like the unwelcome guest it is: release it, exhale it away, and focus on nurturing your own gifts and emotional peace of mind.

CULTIVATE GRATITUDE

When your life is filled with gratitude, you become more spiritually fulfilled. Gratitude makes your experience of the world rich and satisfying. If you want a greater level of contentment and joy in your life, shift your thinking from a focus on what you want to a focus on feeling grateful for what you already have. Look at your life: your body, your environment, and the people around you. There is so much to be grateful for, and the more you recognize this, the better life gets. Gratitude is a sweetly addictive practice, making your life and your world more beautiful.

FOCUS ON YOUR EXHALE AS A WAY OF LETTING GO

Turn your mind toward your breath so that your attention moves inward, away from the distractions of the world around you. Enjoy the fullness of your breath with each inhale. With every exhale, release something that is not serving you: a nagging thought, an item on your to-do list, an anxiety, or a conflict. If the thought you are releasing is particularly persistent, you may need to exhale it again and again, training it to exit your body. You can say to it: *I am letting you go. It is time for you to go. I release you.*

LISTEN WITHOUT JUDGING TO UNDERSTAND THE WORLD

We move through our days making judgments: what to wear, what to eat, how and with whom we wish to spend our time. But consider how we might balance these basic daily judgments with nonjudgmental listening: staying open to the thoughts and ideas of others in order to receive new experiences. We grow as human beings through the reception and assimilation of the unfamiliar. Once we hear what others have to say, we can then decide if and how we want to accept what they are offering. Listening to others' ideas helps us fine-tune our own values and opinions, offering a deeper understanding of ourselves and a more expansive experience of the world.

THE MYTH OF KALI AND RAKTABIJA

The ruthless demon Raktabija was conquering the universe. None of the gods could stop him because he had received a blessing many years earlier that no god or man could kill him. Every time he was wounded on the battlefield, a new demon would arise from each drop of his blood. Soon, his army was immense. The gods called to the ferocious goddess Kali, who was the mother of the universe itself. Kali unrolled her immense tongue along the battlefield, and lapped up all of the blood. Then she latched onto Raktabija, drinking his blood until he fell, lifeless, to the ground. There was nothing Kali could not consume because it had all come from her, since she was the mother of everything that existed. She drew the demonic back into herself to restore balance to the world. Like Kali, you are the mother of your universe. How do you restore your balance?

THE BREATH INVITES EXPANSIVENESS

With each inhale, our lungs fill and our rib cage expands gently outward and upward, similar to an umbrella stretching open. With each exhale, the umbrella is released, allowing us to relax. Because the breath literally expands our upper torso, it can create a feeling of expansiveness within us. This can make us feel more powerful, reminding us that we can always become more open and spacious in our lives simply by breathing. Several times throughout your day today, draw your attention to your breath, noticing whether the experience of your physical expansiveness invites you into a more expansive sense of self.

THE EBB AND FLOW OF YOUR YOGA PRACTICE OVER TIME

Every time you practice yoga, your experience is different from every other time you have practiced yoga. You may still be doing the same poses, and you may still be practicing on the same mat and in the same place. But consider the fact that we grow and change as individuals every day and in every moment. This means that everything is somewhat new each time we do it, including our yoga practice. Over time, you may fall in love with a particular pose or sequence, and then you may fall out of love with it again. You may be drawn to an intense, physically demanding practice, and then your tastes may shift and you prefer a more restorative practice. Like you, your yoga practice can fluctuate and grow in surprising ways over time.

EMBRACE THE RISE
AND FALL OF LIFE

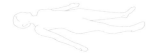

CORPSE POSE
SAVASANA (shah-VAH-sah-nah)

The length of a day, the span of a year, the duration of a life, the blossoming and decay of a flower: your yoga practice mirrors the rhythm of these cyclical natural phenomena. *Savasana*, the Sanskrit name for Corpse Pose, is usually the final pose of a yoga practice session. When we release our bodies into this restful pose, lying on our backs, palms facing up, we acknowledge that everything is born, lives, and passes away. When we take *Savasana*, we acknowledge nature's processes, and join in more fully. We become one with nature through this ritual of *Savasana*. We acknowledge the rise and fall of life and its brevity, its beauty. Each yoga practice is like living a life and completing a cycle; at the end, we rest.

OWN YOUR PAST TO SHAPE YOUR FUTURE

You can't change the past. Whatever has happened to you in your life and whatever choices you have made are now part of who you are. To grow, to move forward, try to own your past. In doing so, you can shape your future. Think of your past as a structure on which you can build. Recognize what did and didn't work, but know that it brought you to where you are right now. Then take what you have learned, refine your building strategy and skills, and transform past events into constructive materials. Begin right now to construct a life you love.

FIND EASE IN
YOUR HEART

To find ease within ourselves, we need to first examine whatever discomfort we may be feeling. Once we know what it stems from, we can begin to manage it. We may be dealing with difficulties in our lives, but we can still find positive, healthy ways in which to live. This begins when we accept the challenges we face. Accepting our challenges doesn't mean that we stop trying to resolve them or to improve. It simply means that we accept that the difficulties are there and that we should not let ourselves lose our peace of mind because of them. In the face of any set of circumstances, remember that there is a sweet place of ease inside us that asks for nothing, offers us acceptance, and allows us to breathe.

MEDITATE ANYWHERE AND EVERYWHERE FOR PEACE OF MIND

You can meditate anywhere and in an infinite number of ways. The more we invite meditation into our daily routine, the more we feel at ease in our lives, and the more smoothly our days unfold. If you are sitting at a desk or in nature, riding a subway car, or waiting for someone, invite yourself to take a few minutes and drop into a meditative state. Begin by turning toward your breath, noticing its rise and fall. Let every exhale release some tension or a thought that is keeping you from a state of ease. Soften your vision and the muscles of your body, and allow yourself to observe your breath for the next few minutes. Meditate anywhere and everywhere for peace of mind.

FIND STILLNESS IN MOVEMENT

When you find yourself moving through a particularly frenzied day, see if you can find, nestled deeply within your center, a small place of stillness. Stillness and movement define each other. There is no meaning to stillness without the concept of motion. Just as we sometimes feel the movement of our hearts and our breath more acutely when our outer bodies are still, and just as we sometimes find a certain tranquility that feels like stillness when we are in motion, so the practice of looking for one within the other will offer you access to your inner sense of balance. Runners or dancers often speak about finding a sort of peaceful suspension within motion. This is because at the center of their constant movement, they have found a deep experience of stillness.

HONOR YOUR ANCESTORS TO HONOR YOUR LIFE

You may be close to your family or you may have a challenging familial situation. But if it weren't for your family and your ancestors, there would be no you, so offer gratitude to them for your life. When you offer gratitude to your ancestors, you tap into the mystery of creation and the culminating sense of you existing in this moment in time, a result of the collective energies of everyone in your lineage who came before you. Your physicality is a result of their mingled chemistry, and who and where you are right now is an outcome of their decisions combined with yours. Honor your ancestors to honor your own life.

MOVE FROM THE FULLNESS OF THE BACK OF YOUR BODY TO SHAPE YOUR FUTURE

The back of your body is behind you. This is obvious, but think of what this means in terms of your experience. You are moving from one place to another. You leave past events and experiences behind to move into the future and shape new ones. The back of your body holds your spine, and we talk about having backbone, meaning that we have determination and firmness in our makeup. When you move from the back of your body, you are moving from this place of firmness and fullness. You use the wisdom gained from past experiences to inform your future.

HIBERNATE IN ORDER
TO CREATE

To be creative, we often need to spend time in creative hibernation. This could involve going for a walk, reading, listening to music, doodling, or quietly finding inspiration in things unrelated to our projects. We may need time to stare off into space or to sit by ourselves and write. We need time for our inner creative impulse to gestate and grow before bringing it out into the world. Creativity cannot be forced, but it can be cultivated. And it is often being cultivated in every calm internal moment that precedes our self-expression. So relax. Daydream. Enjoy your thoughts. And then create.

REVITALIZE YOUR BODY

Prana Mudra (PRAH-nah MOO-drah)
Mudra of Energy

When we are feeling run-down or depleted, we are out of alignment with our *prana*, the Sanskrit word that means both breath and life force. Being sleep-deprived, overworked, or stressed-out can cause this misalignment. To draw ourselves back into a state of revitalization, we need to slow down and begin to engage more deeply with *prana*. Take a seat, and form *Prana Mudra* by touching the tip of your thumb to the tips of your pinkie and ring fingers, extending your middle and index fingers. *Prana Mudra* connects us with our animating life force, helping us regain our vitality.

CHANGE YOUR LIFE NOW

This very moment is your moment of change. As you read this, you have the choice to shift an old dynamic that you don't like and to step into something new. If you want to change your life, begin right now. Choose one small detail to change: give up one habit, do one thing that you've been putting off doing, have that difficult conversation, or make that phone call. Change happens in every moment of our lives, and when you join in, you are part of the greater flow of things. So, choose to participate. Make the small change that has the potential to initiate a cascade of other changes. It only takes one small action. Begin now.

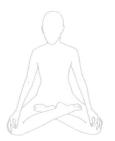

ACKNOWLEDGMENTS

I thank my phenomenally loving parents Hal and Aline Rubin, my beloved sister Jennifer Britton and her family, and the Harwoods, all of whom I adore. Thank you to Emily Stone for referring me to Chronicle, Greg Yamada for your Sanskrit support, and Allan Salkin and Tracy Silver Mazé for your advice. Thank you to Jennifer Unter for your great guidance as my agent, Elizabeth Yarborough for your dedicated editing, and The Writers Room for the physical and mental space. Thank you Michelle Arrington, Harrison Williams, and Luke Hamilton for being spectacular friends, and Leslie Kaminoff, Frank Butler, Jen Resnick, Brenda Villa, Laura Williamson, Gigi Boetto, Janelle Watters-Oliel, Sattva Giacosa, and Brian McKenney for your steadfast support. Thank you, my NYC, Paris, and extended international yoga community for inspiring me, particularly my students. Thank you Douglas Brooks, for being my teacher and friend, for bringing me to India, and for Dr. Gopala Aiyar Sundaramoorthy, because without your Appa, I wouldn't have this yogi heart. *Om Namah Shivaya.*